CAROLE B. WHITENER
MARIE H. KEELING

Illustrations by Jean Bowman

Nutrition Education
for Young Children

strategies and activities

A SPECTRUM BOOK

Prentice-Hall, Inc., Englewood Cliffs, New Jersey 07632

Library of Congress Cataloging in Publication Data

Whitener, Carole B.
  Nutrition education for young children.

  "A Spectrum Book."
  Bibliography: p.
  Includes index.
    1. Children—Nutrition—Study and teaching (Elementary)
2. Children—Nutrition. I. Keeling, Marie H. II. Title.
RJ206.W775 1984   613.2´088054   84-8309
ISBN 0-13-627431-5
ISBN 0-13-627423-4 (pbk.)

For our children, Hank, Lee, and Rebecca

---

1 2 3 4 5 6 7 8 9 10

Editorial/production supervision
by Norma Ledbetter and Chris McMorrow
Cover design © 1984 by Jeannette Jacobs
Manufacturing buyer: Frank Grieco

ISBN 0-13-627431-5

ISBN 0-13-627423-4 {PBK.}

This book is available at a special discount when ordered
in bulk quantities. Contact Prentice-Hall. Inc., General
Publishing Division, Special Sales, Englewood Cliffs, N. J. 07632.

Prentice-Hall International, Inc., *London*
Prentice-Hall of Australia Pty. Limited, *Sydney*
Prentice-Hall Canada Inc., *Toronto*
Prentice-Hall of India Private Limited, *New Delhi*
Prentice-Hall of Japan, Inc., *Tokyo*
Prentice-Hall of Southeast Asia Pte. Ltd., *Singapore*
Whitehall Books Limited, *Wellington, New Zealand*
Editora Prentice-Hall do Brasil Ltda., *Rio de Janeiro*

CONTENTS

PREFACE

This book combines current knowledge of the unique learning styles of infants and young children with practical, lively strategies for effecting positive changes in their nutritional habits and attitudes. The activities were developed to influence the food preferences and practices of even the most finicky eater and to promote the development of basic nutritional concepts in young children.

Although theoretical aspects of nutrition are discussed in this book, the main focus is on implications for practice in programs that serve young children. Strategies for feeding children creatively and well are described. The many recipes for learning include those that allow children to work independently or with small or large groups. Recipes for integrating nutrition education with other curriculum goals; cup cooking; holiday recipes; international recipes; and breakfast, lunch, and snacktime ideas are also given. Additionally, exciting strategies for serving foods and promoting their acceptance are provided.

The activities for learning are "hands-on" activities, designed to help children develop prerequisite knowledge and understandings that lay the foundation for later, more advanced nutrition concepts. Just as language arts and math readiness activities are important prerequisites for reading and mathematical operations, so are experiences with real foods—the kind of food activities we have provided here—prerequisites for higher-level nutrition education. In addition, the activities presented here are just plain good fun for children and their adult caregivers.

Relationships are vital to the success of any nutrition program. For this reason, this book includes numerous ideas for building communication partnerships between those who share the care of young children.

Last, we have included a question and answer chapter that presents issues and questions frequently discussed during our workshops and training sessions. Some of the questions deal with dietary management for children with special problems, and some concern labeling, additives, commercialism, and the more recent issues in nutrition education.

If it is true that we are what we eat, then it follows that young children are what we feed them. Because increasing numbers of infants and young children are spending extended periods away from their parents in the care of others, those others now share the responsibility with parents for providing an optimal nutrition environment.

Since nutrition is the major factor influencing whether or not genetic potential is achieved, the responsibility for feeding children well is awesome. We hope that those who read and use this book will be stimulated to provide sound nutrition programs for young children and that they will seek to influence others who can effect positive changes in the lives of children.

The production of this book would have been impossible without the encouragement and assistance of many people. We are indebted to Ramona Mapp of Tidewater Community College for initiating the project and providing support throughout its development. We are especially grateful to David Shaw, who critically read and reread the manuscript and suggested ways to make the text clearer and more useful, to Nutritionist Katha Root Benton of the Chesapeake Health Department for providing valuable input, and to Margaret Jennings, whose expert word processing skills made the initial drafting of the manuscript less tedious.

Special thanks go to our friends and colleagues of the Humanities Department of Tidewater Community College for their continued interest in our project.

The activities from the book bear the stamp of some of our early mentors and collaborators who have helped to direct and sustain our interest in child development over the years. We especially thank Katharine Kersey of Old Dominion University, whose style of supervision made it possible to be creative.

To our students, who taught us and were kind enough to test our recipes and activities, we are indebted. Most of all, however, we value the assistance given by our families: our parents for providing the nutrients and nurturance we needed during our early years; our husbands, Bill and Henry, without whose endless patience and loving support this book would have been impossible; and our lively children, Rebecca, Hank, and Lee, for stimulating conversation, which provided diversions, insights, and enlightenment to this task.

Figure 1-1 through 1-5 on pages 22 and 23 are provided courtesy of the National Dairy Council.

The recipes on pages 92-101 and page 141 are reprinted from *Snacks to Grow On* by Carole Whitener.

The table on page 24, "Recommended Food Intake for Good Nutrition According to Food Groups and the Average Size of Servings at Different Age Levels," is taken from Vaughan, V.C., McKay R.J., and Berman, R.E., *Nelson Textbook of Pediatrics*, 11th ed., 1979. It is used by permission of W.B. Saunders Co., Philadelphia, PA.

The picture of the Campbell Kids on page 172 is used by permission of the Campbell Soup Company.

Table 8-2 on pages 186-187, "Landmarks of Development," is taken from three tables in Ruth Highberger and Carol Schramm's *Child Development for Day Care Workers,* (Table 1, Landmarks of Infant Development, page 27, Table 2, Landmarks of Toddlerhood Development, page 27, Table 3, Landmarks of Development, page 115). © 1976 by Houghton Mifflin Company. Adapted from Boyd R. McCandless and Ellis Evans, *Children and Youth: Psychosocial Development.*

INTRODUCTION

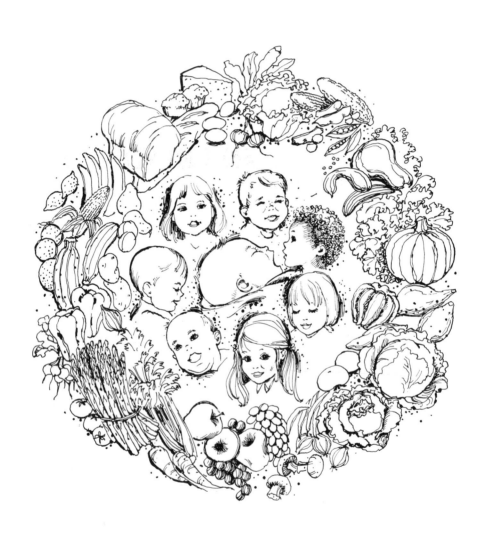

Remarkable changes occur from the moment of conception to the actual birthing of a human being, but the rate of physical, cognitive, and emotional growth is the greatest in the first three years of life. During these first precious years, the one variable that has the most powerful effect upon the growing child is nutrition. Therefore, not only must the mother's nutritional status be adequate to meet the needs of the developing fetus for nine months, but those who are charged with the care and feeding of that child during the early years must also provide an adequate nutritional program.

Child caregivers, teachers, parents, grandparents, cafeteria staff, dietitians, and health care workers all influence the dietary habits and, consequently, the lifelong health of young children. Those who share in the caring for children, who advertise to them, who model eating habits before them, and who otherwise advise or counsel them and their families should be aware of their role in helping children grow into healthy adults.

If nutritional programs provided by these important people are adequate to meet the needs of infants from birth throughout the early years, many learning disabilities, birth defects, childhood diseases, and behavior disorders are prevented. On the other hand, failure to provide good food programs for children can have irreversible and long-lasting consequences.

Only recently have educators and psychologists begun to appreciate the important role that nutrition plays in learning. Efforts to overcome learning deficiencies by "conditioning" or by supplying the child with a stimulating, enriching environment have met with only limited success for the child who has experienced prolonged nutritional insult, particularly during the critical growth period. Although educational techniques such as field trips, filmstrips, and other kinds of environmental stimulation can help a child to compensate for some of the deficiencies suffered as a result of undernutrition, they are never entirely overcome (Cravioto, Robles, 1965).

Furthermore, research on nutrition and growth reveals that undernourished children often grow up to produce children who repeat a similar history with their own children. This cycle often continues for generations. For this reason a major effort has been launched in the United States to intervene. The organization Women, Infants, and Children (WIC), a federally funded intervention program, provides pregnant "at-risk" women and, later, their offspring with nutrition counseling, monitoring, and basic foods that are high in nutritional content. This program also helps children up to age five who are "at risk" to improve their nutritional patterns. This is but one of the many types of programs that can help to break a cycle that might otherwise have negative consequences for generations.

A stimulating child care arrangement, like the Project Head Start program, which provides nutrition counseling for parents and training for caregivers, can augment the gains made by WIC and other intervention programs by helping to ensure that children's nutritional intake remains adequate during their growing years.

Today, many infants and young children are cared for during the working day outside their homes by someone other than their parents. A three-year-old in a child care center who spends eight hours a day, five days a week, beginning at birth, will have spent approximately one-third of his or her life with a caregiver. Obviously, the caregiver will not only be responsible for meeting a large percentage of the child's nutritional requirements but will inadvertently help to influence the child's lifelong dietary habits and food preferences. For this reason, nutritional training is essential for caregivers, especially since we know that caregivers who receive such training are more likely to feed children well than are those who have not participated in nutritional training (Caliendo, Sanjur, 1978).

Because caregivers share with parents the responsibility for ensuring an optimal nutritional environment for young children, they need to be familiar with the nutrient needs of young children and to learn to prepare menus which reflect an understanding of those needs. Furthermore, they must know how to prepare foods to protect their nutritional integrity and to develop strategies for encouraging positive dietary practices in children and their families. They may also need to alter some common dietary practices which have been found to correlate with diseases such as dental caries, obesity, high blood pressure, and cancer.

For a long time, those who work with young children have looked for meaningful ways to include nutrition education in the early learning experiences of young children. Typically, activities in resource books have required children to memorize nutrition facts without regard for the young child's need to conceptualize underlying nutrition principles. These popular rote activities, mostly centered around learning the Basic Four Food guide, have not been found to influence young children's dietary practices. Their value is extremely limited, because they do not promote positive changes in the eating habits of young children, nor do they facilitate the development of nutrition concepts.

Nutrition Education for Young Children: Strategies and Activities offers a different approach. It is not a watered-down version of upper-level nutrition education. This book takes into account that, since young children are not merely miniature versions of adults or older children, their thinking and learning styles are different. Therefore, the activities to promote learning and to influence their behaviors must also be different and reflect an understanding of the developmental levels of the children for whom they are planned.

Providing an adequate nutrition program for young children is an awesome responsibility when one considers the consequences of poor dietary practice, neglect, or indifference. It should be remembered that, since all experiences with food are "learning experiences," each person who is involved in preparing and serving food to children is an active participant in their nutritional education. Most often, the dietary practices of adults in the present become the lifelong dietary habits of children and profoundly affect their futures. Good nutritional habits formed in the early years lay the foundation upon which human potential is built.

chapter one

planning and

preparing **MEALS**

in programs
for young children

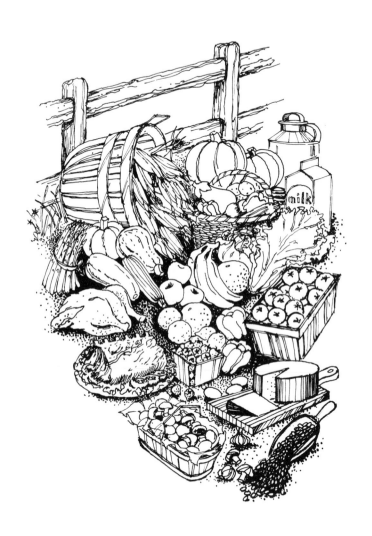

OBJECTIVES

After reading this chapter the reader will be able to:

- Identify each of the nutrient categories, their food sources, benefits, and disease deficiency claims.
- Plan a balanced 4-week cycle of menus that will supply the nutrients required by children at various age levels.
- Discuss factors that influence the food choices of young children.
- Develop a sanitary food management system.

The energy expended by young children at play is a source of amazement to any adult who is charged with the responsibility of keeping up with them. New skills like bouncing, climbing, swinging, marching up and down stairs, and "riding a horsie into town" on the ankles of willing adults are practiced tirelessly and with enthusiasm. Because their energy expenditure is so great and their growth rates so rapid, meeting the nutritional requirements of the growing, perpetually moving child is critical.

Six categories of nutrients are required daily in balanced portions to provide the necessary energy, to promote growth of new cells and tissues, to repair old or injured tissue, and to perform specialized functions like the maintenance of proper levels of body fluids in the growing child. These six categories—protein, carbohydrates, fats, vitamins, minerals, and water—are all found in a well-balanced diet. A variety of factors such as age, activity level, growth rate, and health influence how much of each nutrient is needed by individual children. Adults who are responsible for feeding children need to be aware of how children's nutrient requirements change from day to day and year to year, so they can plan appropriate menus.

MEETING THE NUTRIENT REQUIREMENTS
OF INFANTS AND YOUNG CHILDREN

A glance at Tables 1-1 and 1-2 reveals the recommended daily allowances (RDA) of protein, vitamins, and minerals for children and normal adults.

TABLE 1-1 RDA (Recommended Daily Allowances),[a] Revised 1980
Designed for the Maintenance of Good Nutrition for Healthy American Population

	Age (years)	Weight (kg)	Weight (lb)	Height (cm)	Height (in)	Protein (g)	FAT-SOLUBLE VITAMINS Vitamin A (μRE)[b]	FAT-SOLUBLE VITAMINS Vitamin D (μg)[c]	FAT-SOLUBLE VITAMINS Vitamin E (mg α-TE)
Infants	0.0–0.5	6	13	60	24	kg × 22	420	10	3
	0.5–1.0	9	20	71	28	kg × 2.0	400	10	4
Children	1–5	13	29	90	35	23	400	10	5
	4–6	20	44	112	44	30	500	10	6
	7–10	28	62	132	52	34	700	10	7
Males	11–14	45	99	157	62	45	1000	10	8
	15–18	66	145	176	69	56	1000	10	10
	19–22	70	154	177	70	56	1000	7.5	10
	23–50	70	154	178	70	56	1000	5	10
	51 +	70	154	178	70	56	1000	5	10
Females	11–14	46	101	157	62	46	800	10	8
	15–18	55	120	163	64	46	800	10	8
	19–22	55	120	163	64	44	800	7.5	8
	23–50	55	120	163	64	44	800	5	8
	51 +	55	120	163	64	44	800	5	8
Pregnant:						+ 30	+ 200	+ 5	+ 2
Lactating						+ 20	+ 400	+ 5	+ 3

[a]The allowances are intended to provide for individual variations among most normal persons as they live in the United States under usual environmental stresses. Diets should be based on a variety of common foods in order to provide other nutrients for which human requirements have been less well defined.
[b]Retinol equivalents one retinol equivalent = one μg retinol or 6 μg β carotene.
[c]As cholecalciferol, 10 μg cholecalciferol = 400 IU of vitamin D.
[d]α-tocopherol equivalents, one mg d-αtocopherol = one α-TE.
[e]One NE (niacin equivalent) is equal to one mg of niacin or 60 mg of dietary tryptophan.
[f]The folacin allowances refer to dietary sources as determined by *Lactobacillus cases* assay after treatment with enzymes (conjugases) to make polyglutamyl forms of the vitamin available to the test organism.
[g]The recommended dietary allowance for vitamin B_{12} in infants is based on average concentration of the vitamin in human milk. The allowances after weaning are based on energy intake (as recommended by the American Academy of Pediatrics) and consideration of other factors, such as intestinal absorption.
[h]The increased requirement during pregnancy cannot be met by the iron content of habitual American diets nor by the existing iron stores of many women; therefore the use of 30–60 mg of supplemental iron is recommended. Iron needs during lactation are not substantially different from those of nonpregnant women, but continued supplementation of the mother for 2–3 months after parturition is advisable in order to replenish stores depleted by pregnancy.
Source: Recommended Daily Dietary Allowances, Revised 1980, Food and Nutrition Board, National Academy of Sciences, National Research Council, Washington, D.C.

TABLE 1–1 (Continued)

WATER-SOLUBLE VITAMINS							MINERALS					
Vita-min C (mg)	Thia-min (mg)	Ribo-flavin (mg)	Niacin (mg NE)[e]	Vita-min B-6 (mg)	Fola-cin[f] (µg)	Vitamin B-12[g] (µg)	Cal-cium (mg)	Phos-phorus (mg)	Mag-nesium (mg)	Iron (mg)	Zinc (mg)	Iodine (µg)
35	0.3	0.4	6	0.3	30	0.5	360	240	50	10	3	40
35	0.5	0.6	8	0.6	45	1.5	540	360	70	15	5	50
45	0.7	0.8	9	0.9	100	2.0	800	800	150	15	10	70
45	0.9	1.0	11	1.3	200	2.5	800	800	200	10	10	90
45	1.2	1.4	16	1.6	300	3.0	800	800	250	10	10	120
50	1.4	1.6	18	1.8	400	3.0	1200	1200	350	18	15	150
60	1.4	1.7	18	2.0	400	3.0	1200	1200	400	18	15	150
60	1.5	1.7	19	2.2	400	3.0	800	800	350	10	15	150
60	1.4	1.6	18	2.2	400	3.0	800	800	350	10	15	150
60	1.2	1.4	16	2.2	400	3.0	800	800	350	10	15	150
50	1.1	1.3	15	1.8	400	3.0	1200	1200	300	18	15	150
60	1.1	1.3	14	2.0	400	3.0	1200	1200	300	18	15	150
60	1.1	1.3	14	2.0	400	3.0	800	800	300	18	15	150
60	1.0	1.2	13	2.0	400	3.0	800	800	300	18	15	150
60	1.0	1.2	13	2.0	400	3.0	800	800	300	10	15	150
+20	+0.4	+0.3	+2	+0.6	+400	+1.0	+400	+400	+150	h	+5	+25
+40	+0.5	+0.5	+5	+0.5	+100	+1.0	+400	+400	+150	h	+10	+50

One should keep in mind that these are only *recommended* allowances, since the actual amount of each nutrient required may vary from individual to individual.

Calories

Three of the nutrients—protein, carbohydrates, and fats—provide the calories or energy needed for development. Everything children do requires calories: playing, sitting, crying, sleeping, and even digesting food. And infants require considerably more calories per body weight than older children or adults.

Individual activity patterns greatly influence the energy intake needs of children. For example, infants who play on the floor, which encourages exploratory play, or who are by nature active, may require more calories than children who are confined to cribs or who are by nature less active. It is important to maintain an energy balance; the amount of energy expended should equal the caloric intake. This balance is necessary to maintain normal weight (see Table 1–3).

PROTEIN

The protein requirement for infants (about half of the adult requirement until age three) is relatively higher per body weight than that for adults. An adequate supply of protein is necessary to meet the demands of rapidly

TABLE 1-2 Estimated Safe and Adequate Daily Dietary Intakes of Selected Vitamins and Minerals

| | Age (years) | VITAMINS[a] | | |
		Vitamin K (µg)	Biotin (µg)	Pantothenic Acid (mg)
Infants	0–0.5	12	35	2
	0.5–1	10–20	50	3
Children	1–3	15–30	65	3
and	4–6	20–40	85	3–4
Adolescents	7–10	30–60	120	4–5
	11 +	50–100	100–200	4–7
Adults		70–140	100–200	4–7

| | Age (years) | TRACE ELEMENTS[b] | | | | | |
		Copper (mg)	Man-ganese (mg)	Fluoride (mg)	Chromium (mg)	Selenium (mg)	Molyb-denum (mg)
Infants	0–0.5	0.5–0.7	0.5–0.7	0.1–0.5	0.01–0.04	0.01–0.04	0.03–0.06
	0.5–1	0.7–1.0	0.7–1.0	0.2–1.0	0.02–0.06	0.02–0.06	0.04–0.08
Children	1–3	1.0–1.5	1.0–1.5	0.5–1.5	0.02–0.08	0.02–0.08	0.05–0.1
and	4–6	1.5–2.0	1.5–2.0	1.0–2.5	0.03–0.12	0.03–0.12	0.06–0.15
Adolescents	7–10	2.0–2.5	2.0–3.0	1.5–2.5	0.05–0.2	0.05–0.2	0.10–0.3
	11 +	2.0–3.0	2.5–5.0	1.5–2.5	0.05–0.2	0.05–0.2	0.15–0.5
Adults		2.0–3.0	2.5–5.0	1.5–4.0	0.05–0.2	0.05–0.2	0.15–0.5

| | Age (years) | ELECTROLYTES | | |
		Sodium (mg)	Potassium (mg)	Chloride (mg)
Infants	0–0.5	115–350	350–925	275–700
	0.5–1	250–750	425–1275	400–1200
Children	1–3	325–975	550–1650	500–1500
and	4–6	450–1350	775–2325	700–2100
Adolescents	7–10	600–1800	1000–3000	925–2775
	11 +	900–2700	1525–4575	1400–4200
Adults		1100–3300	1875–5625	1700–5100

[a]Because there is less information on which to base allowances, these figures are not given in the main table of RDA and are provided here in the form of ranges of recommended intakes.
[b]Since the toxic levels for many elements may be only several times usual intakes, the upper levels for the trace elements given in this table should not be habitually exceeded.
Source: Recommended Dietary Allowances, Revised 1980, Food and Nutrition Board, National Academy of Sciences, National Research Council, Washington, D.C.

growing body and muscle tissue in infants and young children. Protein is an important energy source and is vital to brain growth and functioning.

Proteins are found in varying amounts in all foods. Meats, however, provide the only source of complete protein—that is, protein containing all of the "essential" amino acids needed for the body to utilize protein. Vegetables and fruits are sources of incomplete protein: They lack one or more of the essential amino acids that must be present for protein to be utilized by the body. For this reason, vegetarians must combine vegetable, grains,

TABLE 1-3   Mean Heights and Weights and Recommended Energy Intake

Category	AGE (Years)	WEIGHT (kg)	WEIGHT (lb)	HEIGHT (cm)	HEIGHT (in.)	ENERGY NEEDS (WITH RANGE) (kcal)	ENERGY NEEDS (WITH RANGE) (MJ)
Infants	0.0-0.5	6	13	60	24	kg × 115 (95-145)	kg × .48
	0.5-1.0	9	20	71	28	kg × 105 (80-135)	kg × .44
Children	1-3	13	29	90	35	1300 (900-1800)	5.5
	4-6	20	44	112	44	1700 (1300-2300)	7.1
	7-10	28	62	132	52	2400 (1650-3300)	10.1
Males	11-14	45	99	157	62	2700 (2000-3700)	11.3
	15-18	66	145	176	69	2800 (2100-3900)	11.8
	19-22	70	154	177	70	2900 (2500-3300)	12.2
	23-50	70	154	178	70	2700 (2300-3100)	11.3
	51-75	70	154	178	70	2400 (2000-2800)	10.1
	76 +	70	154	178	70	2050 (1650-2450)	8.6
Females	11-14	46	101	157	62	2200 (1500-3000)	9.2
	15-18	55	120	163	64	2100 (1200-3000)	8.8
	19-22	55	120	163	64	2100 (1700-2500)	8.8
	23-50	55	120	163	64	2000 (1600-2400)	8.4
	51-75	55	120	163	64	1800 (1400-2200)	7.6
	76 +	55	120	163	64	1600 (1200-2000)	6.7
Pregnancy						+ 300	
Lactation						+ 500	

Source: *Nutrition for the Growing Years,* by Margaret McWilliams, third edition, © 1980 by John Wiley & Sons, Inc., p. 48. Reprinted by permission of John Wiley & Sons, Inc.

and legumes carefully to ensure that all the essential amino acids are present if their protein needs are to be met.

The quality of protein that is consumed surpasses the quantity in the degree of importance. For example, human milk contains less protein than cow's milk, but most of the protein in human milk can be digested and maintained by the infant, while a high percentage of the protein in cow's milk is bypassed and eliminated. However, cow's milk, human milk, and prepared formulas all contain the essential amino acids that are necessary for optimal growth and development (*Pediatric Nutrition Handbook*, 1979).

CARBOHYDRATES

Carbohydrates are an important source of energy. When they are available in sufficient amounts to meet the body's energy requirements, protein, which is needed for growth and muscle and tissue maintenance, is spared. Carbohydrates also help the body metabolize fats, provide glucose for brain functioning, and provide cellulose (bulk) or fiber to help eliminate wastes.

Except for milk and milk products, nearly all the carbohydrates we consume are from plant sources. They consist of all the common sugars, starches, pectin, and cellulose. Simple carbohydrates, such as sugars like honey, glucose, corn syrup, lactose, date sugar, turbinado sugar, maltose, fructose, sucrose, and dextrins, contain little more than calories and are lacking in other nutrients. However, when simple carbohydrates occur naturally in foods rather than added as sweeteners, a good ratio exists between calories and nutrients. Complex carbohydrates are found in beans, peas,

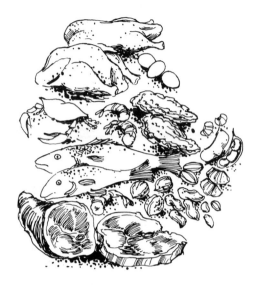

nuts, and whole-grain cereals and breads. These provide essential nutrients and fiber needed for digestion.

FATS

Like protein and carbohydrates, fat offers a third supply of energy. It contributes more than twice as many calories per gram as carbohydrates. This is significant, because fat provides the small child who has a limited volume capacity with the calories that are needed for rapid growth and high levels of activity. Energy from this source also helps to spare the body's protein.

Fats are an important addition to the diet of very young children, for they are the only source of an essential fatty acid, linoleic acid, which is necessary for optimum growth and healthy skin. Scaly skin, smaller than normal cell membranes, and stunted growth have been associated with low-fat diets in young children. Therefore, fat-free diets and skim milk should be avoided for most healthy children under the age of three. Children from families with a history of obesity or high serum cholesterol levels, however, may need to pursue this issue further with a dietary counselor.

Fat is found in almost equal amounts in human and cow's milk. Eggs, organ meats (like liver), meat, cream, butter, and coconut oil are all sources of fats. Saturated fats are derived from animal sources. It is thought that Americans, in general, consume more saturated fats than good health mandates.[1] Replacing some of them with polyunsaturated fats (vegetable oils) and reducing the overall consumption of fats are considered to be sensible practices.

[1]*Nutrition and Your Health: Dietary Guidelines for Americans* is a publication by the U.S. Department of Agriculture, Home and Garden Bulletin No. 232. It can be ordered from: Supertendent of Documents, U.S. Government Printing Office, Washington, D.C. 20402.

Minerals and Vitamins

Table 1-4 provides a list of minerals and vitamins, their food sources, and deficiency disease claims. Since they are the body's protectors and are necessary for normal tissue and organ functioning, they must be regularly available in adequate amounts in children's diets. Some of them, however, are too often in short supply.

MINERALS

Minerals are inorganic chemical compounds or elements. A full-term infant derives its store of minerals during the last trimester of gestation. Minerals are only required in small amounts by the body. Some minerals, called *trace minerals,* are needed in such small portions that weight assignment for daily requirement is impossible. However, this does not mean they are of little value to the body. Mineral deficiencies are found in the United States as they are in most other countries. Serving children a variety of foods ensures them of meeting daily mineral requirements.

Iron. A three-month supply of iron is normally present at birth. It has been generally thought that the newborn child of a well-nourished mother should have an adequate supply of iron and be able to thrive on breast milk until iron-fortified cereals can be added to the diet. However, Foman et al. (1979) and the American Academy of Pediatrics now recommend a daily supplement of 7 milligrams of iron for breast-fed infants.

Infants who are fed on commercially prepared formulas that are iron fortified, however, require no additional iron supplements. Cereals that are added to the diet when the infant is five or six months old should be iron fortified, and the infant should eat them daily until about eighteen months old.

As a child grows, iron requirements decrease. Even so, young children frequently experience iron deficiency anemia, a serious condition requiring the attention of a health care professional. It should not be ignored, nor should home remedies replace medical attention.

Characteristically, the condition slows the intake of oxygen to the brain and has a negative effect on mental functioning. Although the condition does not lower intelligence, a shorter attention span has been noted in young children who suffer from it. They have been seen to manipulate objects with no apparent intent, and their play, in general, appears random and disorganized. They also characteristically show a limited ability to concentrate, are generally listless, sleepy, lack energy, have a lower resistance to infection, and are pale in appearance. All of these symptoms interfere with school functioning and result in a decreased interest in school activity.

Unfortunately, foods are rich in iron—nuts, dark vegetables, organ meats, and whole-grain cereals, are among the least favorite of children. Therefore, the adult needs to find ingenious ways of adding these foods

TABLE 1-4 Minerals, Vitamins, Food Sources, and Disease Deficiency Claims

SOME MINERALS RECOGNIZED AS NUTRITIONALLY IMPORTANT IN YOUNG CHILDREN			
Minerals	Functions	Disease Claims	Sources[a]
Calcium	Bone and tooth formation. Regulation of heart and other muscle contraction. Transmission of nerve impulses.	Poor growth. Bowed legs. Poor quality teeth.	Milk, cheese, yogurt, collard, kale, mustard, turnip greens, small fish with bones.
Chromium	Necessary for production of insulin.	Impaired glucose tolerance. Slow weight gain in malnourished infants.	Meats, whole-grain cereal and bread.
Copper	Promotes iron absorption. Contains enzymes required for energy. Maintains blood vessels and nervous system.	Anemia. Rupture of the major arteries.	Meat, eggs, nuts, shellfish.
Iodine	Formation of the hormone thyroxin, which regulates normal metabolism.	Goiters.	Iodized salt, seafood, processed foods.
Iron	Combines with protein to form hemoglobin. Increases resistance to infection.	Anemia, fatigue, listlessness.	Liver, prune juice, meat, legumes, molasses.
Magnesium	Regulates cardiac and skeletal muscles. Aids nervous tissue function.	Convulsions. Muscle dysfunction.	Milk, whole grains, nuts, fresh green vegetables.
Potassium	Maintenance of acid-base balance. Catalyst for protein formation. Necessary for muscle contraction.	Renal diseases. Muscular weakness.	Oranges, bananas, grapefruit, fish, green beans.
Phosphorus	Necessary for bone and teeth formation.	(Deficiency is not likely to occur.)	Meats, milk, cheese, fruits, whole grains
Sodium	Maintains osmotic pressure (fluid). Aids in the transmission of nerve impulses.	Weakness. Fainting. May contribute to hypertension.	Table salt, processed foods.
Zinc	Required for optimum growth. A component of enzyme systems.	Impaired growth. wound healing. Reduced sense of taste.	Milk, whole-grain cereals, oysters, clams, meats.

VITAMINS NECESSARY FOR PROMOTING GROWTH AND DEVELOPMENT

Vitamins	Functions	Disease Claims	Sources[a]
Fat-soluble Vitamins			
Vitamin A[b] (Retinol)	Vision. Growth. Helps keep skin smooth. Aids in keeping infection from mucous membranes.	Night blindness. Dry, itchy skin. Infections.	Butter, margarine, egg yolks, fruit, dark green vegetables, carrots, sweet potatoes.
Vitamin D[b] (Calciferol)	Aids the body in absorbing and utilizing calcium and phosphorus.	Rickets. Osteomalacia.	Natural source—sunshine, which converts vitamin D when in contact with the skin. Vitamin-fortified milk, cheese.
Vitamin E (Antisterility vitamin)	Antioxidant. Malabsorption and muscle defects.	No definite deficiency; however many claims accompany low consumption, such as boils, colitis, epilepsy, ulcers, and stroke, to name a few.	Leafy green vegetables, oils, nuts, liver.
Vitamin K[b] (Coagulation vitamin)	Blood clotting.	Hemorrhage.	Dark green leafy vegetables, egg yolk, soybean oil, liver.
Water-soluble Vitamins			
Vitamin B$_1$ (Thiamine)	Helps release energy from carbohydrates, protein, and fat. Aids in neural functions. Tissue respiration and growth.	Beriberi (characterized by numbness of feet and toes, leg cramps). Retarded growth. Sensitivity to pain.	Wheat germ, whole-grain cereals, nuts, legumes, meat, fish.
Vitamin B$_2$ (Riboflavin)	Helps cellular respiration. Metabolizes carbohydrates, proteins, and fats.	Stunted growth in infants. Cracks at the corners of mouth and mouth sores (cheilosis). Dermatitis.	Milk, cheese, meat, asparagus, broccoli, whole-wheat and enriched bread and cereals.
Vitamin B$_3$[b] (Niacin)	Aids in cells using other nutrients. Helps tissue oxidation. Healthy nervous system.	Pellegra, sometimes referred to as the 3 D's—diarrhea, dermatitis, and dementia. Weakness. Poor appetite. Confusion.	Meat, peanut butter, fish, enriched bread and cereals.
Vitamin B$_6$ (Pyridoxine)	Metabolizes protein and helps the release of protein energy. Aids in the production of antibodies.	Mental disorders. Skin inflammation and low hemoglobin concentration.	Wheat germ, whole-wheat grains and cereals, meats, bananas, legumes, greens, potatoes.

TABLE 1-4 (Continued)

Vitamins	Functions	Disease Claims	Sources[a]
Vitamin B₅ (Pantothenic acid)	Essential as an energy releaser from food.	Mental disorders, depression, fatigue, mental illness. Decreased antibody formation.	Organ meats, eggs, milk, wheat bran, wheat germ, most foods.
Vitamin B₁₂ (Cobalamine)	Blood cell formation Produces insulators surrounding nerve cells.	Anemia. Irreversible neurological damage.	Organ meats, poultry, fish, milk, cheese, eggs.
Folacin[b] (Folic acid)	Cell growth, maturation and reproduction. Synthesis of DNA.	Similar blood changes as vitamin B₁₂ deficiency.	Spinach and other dark green, leafy vegetables, also mushrooms, liver, and kidney.
Vitamin C[b] (Ascorbic acid)	Formation of collagen, the cementing material that holds body cells together. Protection against infection. Helps heal wounds and broken bones. Promotes calcification of teeth and keeps gums healthy.	Scurvy (listlessness and pain in joints). Tooth and gum diseases. Hemorrhages under the skin. Lowered resistance to infection.	Citrus fruits, strawberries, tomatoes, potatoes, cabbage, green leafy vegetables.
Biotin	Releases energy from glucose. Produces antibodies.	Deficiency unheard of in humans. Few claims made.	Eggs, organ meats, milk, sardines, cauliflower.

[a]The first source listed is the primary source for obtaining the mineral or vitamins.
[b]These vitamins have been attributed to potential toxicities in the body. Vitamin supplements should be avoided except by a physician's recommendation.

to the menu. It would also be helpful to combine foods which have a high iron content with foods which are rich sources of vitamin C (fruit juices, broccoli, fruit) to aid iron absorption. Protein foods also combine with iron to make hemoglobin.

Iron-rich foods are frequently inadequately represented in menus for young children. Williams et al. (1977) found in a review of forty-eight child care center programs that, although the caregivers were able to include sources of most vitamins in their menus, they often had difficulty planning menus that provided the RDA for iron.

Calcium and Phosphorus. Calcium and phosphorus are particularly important for child growth and development. Calcium is necessary to support the rapid growth of the skeletal structure and teeth, to aid in blood clotting, and help nerve transmission. Phosphorus plays an important role in the metabolism and is also a structural component of teeth and bones. These minerals are interdependent and are present in adequate amounts in both cow's and human milk. Milk products, dried beans, fish, and dark green leafy vegetables are additional sources of phosphorus.

Fluoride. Each mineral is usually found in sufficient quantities in food with the exception of fluoride. Fluoride, in most cases, is added to the tap water when the natural artesian well supply is inadequate. This practice, along with the addition of fluoride to toothpaste which commands about 80 percent of the market, has cut tooth decay by an astounding one-third during this past decade. Fluoridated water is still a relatively new concept, and many people are not protected by it. Therefore, it is recommended that infants living in areas where the fluoride content of the water is less then 0.3 ppm, a fluoride supplement of approximately .25 mg per day is needed.[2]

In some areas of the country the levels of fluoride in the artesian supply is excessive. Unless other provisions are made for cooking and drinking water, the excessive fluoride can produce florosis, a brown mottling of the teeth.

VITAMINS

The word *vitamin* is derived from the combination of two words—*vital* and *amine*. The word *vital* indicates the importance of the compounds, and the word *amine* is derived from the fact that most of the vitamins contain ammonia. Deficiencies of most vitamins are rare in the United States. However, even a slight vitamin deficiency in children has been found to be more devastating than one in adults. In most cases, a slight deficiency may claim a problem without an extreme disorder. Symptoms of deficiency usually disappear when moderate amounts of the vitamin are prescribed by a physician. The best way to safeguard children against vitamin undernutrition is to serve them a variety of wholesome foods.

Vitamins can be divided into two categories—water-soluble and fat-soluble. Water-soluble vitamins (C and B vitamins) that are not utilized by the body are excreted. They must be replaced by providing children with foods containing them several times daily. Since children's diets are likely to be deficient in one or more of the B vitamins, be sure to check Table 1-4 for rich sources of them and include them, along with vitamin C sources, in your daily menu.

Fat-soluble vitamins (A, D, E, and K) are stored in body tissues. When they are consumed in excessive amounts, particularly in the form of pills, they can become toxic agents.

Foods that are rich in carotene, which our bodies convert to vitamin A (deep yellow and dark green vegetables are sources of carotene) should be given to young children regularly. Since children frequently reject these vitamin A-rich foods, adults must find clever ways of making them appealing to children. For example, try shredding raw spinach into a salad rather than serving it cooked. Squash too is more acceptable with a child-made dip or as a "veggie-pop."

It is important to remember that vitamins are not medicine but are

---

[2]S. J. Foman and others, *Recommendations for Feeding Normal Infants,* DHEW Publication No. (HSA) 79-5108 (Washington, D.C.: U.S. Government Printing Office, 1979).

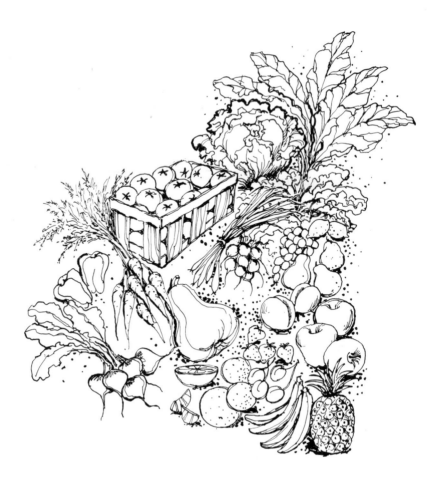

found in adequate amounts in foods that are well prepared and served in balanced portions. There are no known advantages to consuming mega-doses of any nutrient for most healthy people, and the danger of toxic over-dose from pills is real.

Water

Water plays an important role in meeting nutritional needs. It is a universal solvent. After nutrients have been digested, water transports them to cells and, in turn, carries out cellular wastes. Water also helps to regulate body temperature, lubricate the joints, and provide some needed minerals.

The human body is 55 to 65 percent water. For children to maintain a healthy fluid level, water must be consumed daily in the form of juice, soup, hot or cold beverages, or ideally in its pure form. Dehydration can be fatal for small children. During hot weather or when there is a rise in body temperature due to an illness, young children's water requirements increase.

PLANNING MENUS
FOR YOUNG CHILDREN

Knowing the nutrient requirements of young children is an important first step in meal planning. But organizing this information into a workable system for meal planning is a real challenge. It is little wonder that, for many people, meal planning consists of a trip to the pantry or to the grocery store where menu items are selected haphazardly.

In most family day care homes, as in the homes of many children, menus reflect the food preferences and whimsical fancies of the adults in charge. Too often this is the case in day care centers also. If certain foods are avoided or if adults have a narrow range of preferences, the foods they present to children will be limited in variety. If adult diets lack nutrients, and research suggests that the diets of at least 50 percent of the population are low in one or more vital nutrient (Cott, 1972), then it is likely that the children they serve will also lack important nutrients, nutrients children need for growth. It is important, therefore, to plan and evaluate menus carefully to ensure that a wide range of foods containing a balance of nutrients is presented to children daily. Menu items should not be governed by the preferences of the adults in charge.

The Basic Four Food Plan

The Basic Four Food guide was developed in 1954 for the purpose of simplifying menu planning. In this plan, food is grouped into four categories: (1) milk and dairy products, (2) meat and meat products, (3) fruits and vegetables, and (4) breads and cereals. Recently a fifth group called "others" was added to cover foods that were too nutritionally deficient to be included in the basic four plan. This grouping makes the task of menu planning a less overwhelming task for the novice.

Each group emphasizes one or more major nutrients. For example, the members of the milk group contain much more calcium than most other foods. Members of the meat group are easily remembered for their high protein content. The foods in the fruit and vegetable group contain vitamins A and C, and the grain group is known for its ready supply of carbohydrates and B vitamins.

MILK GROUP

With each food group, a recommended number of daily servings is indicated. The milk group, however, specifies not only the number of servings needed, but the amount that should be served to each age group. Infants, young children, and teenagers, who grow at a rapid rate, naturally require more calcium for bone growth than adults; therefore, they will need more servings. Adults, however, are encouraged to consume at least two servings of milk or milk products a day. (See Figure 1-1.)

FIGURE 1-1

milk
Group

	2 Servings/Adults 4 Servings/Teenagers 3 Servings/Children
Calcium Riboflavin (B₂) Protein	Foods made from milk contribute part of the nutrients supplied by a serving of milk.

Calcium
Riboflavin (B₂)
Protein

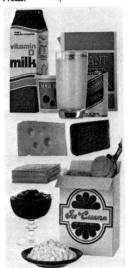

FIGURE 1-2

meat
Group

Protein
Niacin
Iron
Thiamin (B₁)

2 Servings

Dry beans and peas,
soy extenders, and nuts
combined with animal
protein (meat, fish,
poultry, eggs, milk,
cheese) or grain protein
can be substituted for
a serving of meat.

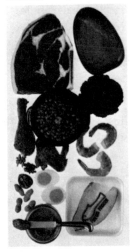

MEAT GROUP

Only two servings of meat or meat products are required daily according to this plan. At first glance, this may appear to be an inadequate amount of protein; however, a look at Table 1-1 reveals that for a young child, only 23 to 30 grams of protein is needed daily. One boiled egg provides the child with 7 grams of protein, meeting almost one-fourth of the daily requirement. If a breakfast sausage and a cup of milk are served with the egg, approximately 19 more grams of protein are added. With this breakfast, the child will have consumed all of the proteins needed for the entire day. Perhaps a better plan would be to spread out the high protein foods during the course of the day. Most Americans consume twice the amount of protein their bodies need. (See Figure 1-2.)

FRUIT AND VEGETABLE, BREAD AND CEREAL GROUPS

The fruit and vegetable and the bread and cereal groups require four servings from each group every day. Because vitamins C and B found in fruits, vegetables, and whole grains are water soluble, they must be consumed frequently throughout the day. (See Figures 1-3 and 1-4.)

The serving sizes for each of the food groups are outlined in Table 1-5. Serving sizes should vary, of course, in response to individual energy requirements.

FIGURE 1-3

Fruit- _{4 Servings}
Vegetable
Group

**Vitamins A
and C** | Dark green, leafy, or orange vegetables and fruit are recommended 3 or 4 times weekly for vitamin A. Citrus fruit is recommended daily for vitamin C.

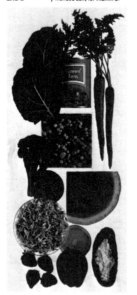

FIGURE 1-4

Grain | 4 Servings
Group | Whole grain, fortified, or enriched grain products are recommended.

**Carbohydrate
Thiamin (B₁)
Iron
Niacin**

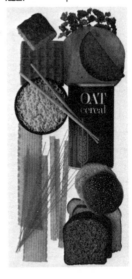

FIGURE 1-5

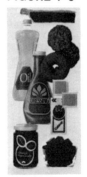

Foods and condiments
such as these complement
but do not replace foods
from the four groups.
Amounts should be deter-
mined by individual
caloric needs.

Others

**Carbohydrate
Fats**

For many years, the basic four has served as an adequate guide to menu planning. However, changes in culture and life styles, the results of new disease research, and the introduction of a wide range of new foods have served to complicate its use for today's menu planner.

An increasing body of research linking diet and certain diseases seems to indicate a need for consuming larger amounts of some foods while eating less of others. The Basic Four plan does not discriminate between the foods contained within each category in terms of which should be consumed more or less frequently. It does not, for example, distinguish between those foods in each group which are high in calories, fats, simple carbohydrates, and salt. A meal of poultry, spinach, skimmed milk, whole-wheat bread, and fruit and a meal consisting of a wiener on a white bun, french fries, and a milk shake could both be planned by following the Basic Four guide. Clearly, they both follow the plan, but they are obviously not nutritional equivalents.

If the Basic Four plan is to be used as a guide, it should be used discriminately. Menu planners should be aware that many breakfast cereals, some of which contain as much as 55 percent sugar, are not the nutritional equivalent of whole-grain cereals; likewise, potato chips are not nutritionally equivalent to boiled potatoes, nor are fruit drinks substitutes for fruit juice.

The introduction to the market of fabricated foods whose nutritional composition is often not consistent with the foods they mimic compounds

TABLE 1-5 Recommended Food Intake for Good Nutrition According to Food Groups and the Average Size of Servings at Different Age Levels

Food Group	Servings per day	AVERAGE SIZE OF SERVINGS					
		1 year	2-3 years	4-5 years	6-9 years	10-12 years	13-15 years
Milk and cheese (1.5 oz cheese = 1 c[a] milk)	4	½ c	½-¼ c	¼ c	¼-1 c	1 c	1 c
Meat group (protein foods)	3 or more						
Egg		1	1	1	1	1	1 or more
Lean meat, fish, poultry (liver once a week)		2 T[b]	2 T	4 T	2-3 oz (4-6 T)	3-4 oz	4 oz or more
Peanut butter			1 T	2 T	2-3 T	3 T	3 T
Fruits and vegetables							
Vitamin C source (citrus fruits, berries, tomato, cabbage, cantaloupe)	At least 4, including 1 or more (twice as much tomato as citrus)	⅓ c citrus	½ c	½ c	1 medium orange	1 medium orange	1 medium orange
Vitamin A source (green or yellow fruits and vegetables)	1 or more	2 T	3 T	4 T (¼ c)	¼ c	⅓ c	½ c
Other vegetables (potato and legumes, etc.) *or*	2	2 T	3 T	4 T (¼ c)	⅓ c	½ c	¾ c
Other fruits (apple, banana, etc.)		¼ c	⅓ c	½ c	1 medium	1 medium	1 medium
Cereals (whole-grain or enriched)	At least 4						
Bread		½ c	1 slice	1½ slices	1-2 slices	2 slices	2 slices
Ready-to-eat cereals		½ oz	¾ oz	1 oz	1 oz	1 oz	1 oz
Cooked cereal (including macaroni, spaghetti, rice, etc.)		¼ c	⅓ c	½ c	½ c	¾ c	1 c or more
Fats and carbohydrates Butter, margarine mayonnaise, oils: 1 T = 100 calories	To meet calorie needs	1 T	1 T	1 T	2 T	2 T	2-4 T

[a]One cup (1 c) = 8 oz or 240 gm.
[b]T = Tablespoon

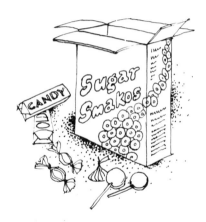

the problem of using the Basic Four plan as a guide. It is increasingly difficult to determine into which categories some foods belong. The menu planner must be alert when selecting from these foods for they frequently contain many calories and few vital nutrients. That is why the National Dairy Council added the fifth category, "others." (See Figure 1-5.)

When choosing menu items from the four basic food groups, it is probably a good idea also to consider the guidelines for health developed in 1980 by the U.S. Department of Agriculture and the Department of Health and Human Services. In the publication, *Nutrition and Your Health: Dietary Guidelines for Americans*, seven goals are stated.[3] The first six are of primary importance to meal planners in programs that serve young children. They are (1) eat a variety of foods; (2) maintain ideal weight; (3) avoid too much fat, saturated fat, and cholesterol; (4) eat foods with adequate starch and fiber; (5) avoid too much sugar; (6) and avoid too much sodium. The seventh goal is: If you drink alcoholic beverages, do so in moderation.

Coordinating Menu Plans to Satisfy Children's Nutrient Requirements

Most menu plans in child care programs include lunch and at least one snack. Some programs serve two snacks and have a breakfast-snack table available for those children who arrive hungry. Regardless of the number of meals or snacks planned, however, they should be coordinated to satisfy the daily nutritional requirements of the children. This can be accomplished by tallying the nutritive values of the foods on the menu plan and checking the totals against the child's RDA (Tables 1-1 and 1-2). A number of publications such as Agriculture Handbook No. 8, *Composition of Foods*, and Agriculture Handbook No. 456, *Nutritive Value of American Goods in Common Units*, contain helpful data on the nutrient content of edible portions of foods. These can be purchased from the Superintendent of Documents, U.S. Government Printing Office, Washington, D.C. 20402.

[3]U.S. Department of Agriculture, Home and Garden Bulletin No. 232 (Washington, D.C.: U.S. Government Printing Office).

According to the Child Care Food Program, lunch should generally include a meat or good source of complete protein and at least two fruits or vegetables, with servings of dark green and leafy or yellow vegetables every other day. Either whole-wheat bread, rice, or enriched noodles should be served daily. The beverage for children over the age of three may be low-fat milk, fortified with vitamin D.

Desserts should also be nutritious. If cookies or cakes are offered, they should be offered rarely, and an effort should be made to boost their nutrient density. Banana bread is more nutritious, for example, than pound cake, and oatmeal cookies offer more nutrients than sugar cookies. Carrot cake and pumpkin breads are good sources of vitamin A, and custards contain calcium. Moreover, fruits should be served frequently for they too make an appealing dessert for young children and are economical, easy to serve, and can be combined in many ways.

Both desserts, if they are served, and snacks should be considered an important part of the daily menu plan, for ideally they offer nutrients and calories that are needed to maintain growth and meet energy requirements.

Planning a Cycle of Menus

Menus should be planned at least four weeks in advance to ensure an adequate nutrient balance. This monthly series should be evaluated closely to determine whether children like the foods you have chosen and to identify other problems that sometimes occur when the food is prepared or served. Initially, some adjustments in the series may be indicated, but once the system is in place, it can be maintained with few changes, except in response to the need for special holiday foods, fluctuations in food prices, or other unforeseen events.

To plan a monthly cycle, first select entrees for twenty days. List them on a chart like the one in Table 1-6. Then, get a calendar and write beside each entree the date on which you will serve it. Develop similar charts for salads, breads, vegetables, and fruits, and coordinate them with the entrees. When you have coordinated the entrees and their accompanying foods to complete a balanced meal for each of the twenty days, you will have

TABLE 1-6 Menu Planning Chart

ENTREES		*DATES*					
Chicken, salad	2/1						
Chicken, fried							
Chicken, baked							
Cottage cheese with fruit							
Fish, baked	1/8						

the information needed for buying in bulk. Now, check the menus against the list of questions provided below.

1. Are the menus nutritionally sound? Does each lunch menu provide one-third or more of the RDA for the children as required by the U.S. Department of Agriculture?

2. Are the snacks chosen to help balance the food plan? Are they nutritious?

3. Are the desserts nutritious? For instance, serving custards; rice pudding; fruit; pumpkin, date, or raisin breads, rather than candy or cookies?

4. Have all means of keeping costs down (without sacrificing quality) been explored? For example, using U.S. Department of Agriculture (USDA) funding; locating available food commodities; bulk buying in cooperation with other centers, caregivers, nursing homes, or schools? Have seasonal foods been considered? Or perhaps the children could become involved in clipping and saving coupons.

5. Have the cultural preferences of the children been considered?

6. Have the dietary practices of the children's families been studied and taken into consideration?

7. Is a food that is unfamiliar to the children planned for snack or mealtime every week or two to help expand their palates?

8. Will each meal be aesthetically pleasing in terms of contrasting temperatures, textures, and colors?

9. Is it possible to prepare everything in the menu plan in the facility and with the utensils that are available? For example, do you have enough oven space to bake breads, casseroles, and meatloaf on the same day? If not, it may be necessary to reschedule some of these items.

10. Have you provided alternatives for children who have food allergies and easy-to-eat food for children who have handicaps?

11. Are failproof, waste-proof recipes available for each item on the menu? Write the U.S. Department of Agriculture, Food and Nutrition Service, Washington, D.C., for *Quantity Recipes for Child Care Centers*, FNS-86, May 1973.

As the menus are prepared and served, mark an asterisk by the items that the children liked the most; mark out those that they refused. Make adjustments in the cycle for the next month to reflect what you learned when the meals were served (Table 1-7 provides an example of a menu that reflects good planning).

Of all the questions outlined above, items 4 and 5, which relate to food preferences, may be the trickiest ones with which to deal. For that reason, a brief discussion of children's food preferences is given below.

TABLE 1-7 Sample Lunch Menus in "Ideas for Administrators"

MENUS		MONDAY	TUESDAY	WEDNESDAY	THURSDAY	FRIDAY
WEEK I		Oven-baked fish Green beans Carrot sticks Cheese biscuits Milk Fresh pear halves	Beef balls Lima beans Tomato wedges Whole-wheat toast strips Milk Stewed prunes	Stewed chicken Buttered noodles Grated carrot-raisin salad Whole-wheat bread with apricot spread Milk Orange slices	Simmered steak Scalloped potatoes English peas Whole-wheat muffins Milk Fresh fruit cup	Ground chicken and egg sandwiches Buttered beets Lettuce pieces and tomato wedges Milk Bananas in gelatin made with orange juice
WEEK II		Meat loaf Buttered carrots and peas Whole-wheat bread and butter Milk Oatmeal muffins	Creamed chicken Buttered rice French green beans Cornbread sticks Milk Seedless grapes	Oven-baked fish Buttered mixed vegetables Whole-wheat toast strips Milk Apple wedges	Toasted cheese sandwich Tomato soup Chopped broccoli Milk Cantaloupe slices	Ham Baked potato with cheese Celery and carrot sticks Whole-wheat toast strips Milk Plain cake with orange sauce
WEEK III		Baked salmon croquettes Scalloped potatoes Okra with tomatoes Whole-wheat bread Milk Apple slices	Meat balls with tomato sauce Green beans Enriched bread and butter Milk Banana bread	Cheese cubes Twice-baked potatoes Buttered beets Cooked spinach with egg slices Milk Vanilla ice cream	Beef stew with peas, carrots, and potatoes French bread pieces Milk Cottage cheese and peach slices	Chicken casserole Buttered broccoli Bran muffins Milk Fresh pineapple and banana slices
WEEK IV		Hard-boiled eggs Green beans with bacon Drop biscuits Milk Orange slices in gelatin	Braised calves liver English peas Perfection salad Whole-wheat toast strips Milk Baked apple	Tuna fish sandwiches Lettuce pieces Buttered summer squash Milk Fresh fruit cup	Creamed chicken Buttered spinach Grated carrot-raisin salad Whole-wheat bread Milk Applesauce	Beef patty and gravy Peas and potatoes Tomato wedges Milk Sliced bananas in orange juice

Reprinted by permission from *The Idea Box*. Washington, D.C.: NAEYC, 1973, p. 31. By the Austin Association for the Education of Young Children © 1973 by the National Association for the Education of Young Children, 1834 Connecticut Ave., N.W., Washington, D.C. 20009.

Food Preferences
of Young Children

No matter how well menus are planned to satisfy the nutrient requirements of young children, if foods are not eaten, all effort is wasted. The fact is that children frequently reject menu items. Since children are really not miniature versions of adults, their food preferences are often hard to predict. They go through stages of liking or disliking certain foods during their growth spurts. By watching their responses to the foods served, however, the menu cycle can be modified to accommodate their tastes while satisfying their nutritional requirements.

The food preferences of young children, most often, but not always, reflect the preferences of their parents; they are more comfortable eating foods with which they are familiar. For this reason it is important to survey parents to determine the foods that are most often served at home. With this practice, menus can be planned to include items that are familiar to the children and reflect the food preferences that are characteristic of their culture (see Table 1-8 for an example of a dietary recall).

However, familiarity is not the only key to acceptance. Sometimes children seem to resist certain foods, no matter how creatively or frequently they are served. This conversation provides an illustration.

"Rebecca, try some spinach. You may like it this time."

"Do I have to?"

"You may be surprised. Sometimes we find that we like things after

TABLE 1-8 Food Intake Recording Form
to Be Filled Out by Parents

Dear Parents,

To help us plan an adequate nutrition program for your child, we need your help. Kindly fill out this form and return it with your child in one week. Try to record all foods eaten for breakfast, dinner, and snacks each day in the spaces provided on the form.

Name of child _____

WEEKDAY	SNACKS	BREAKFAST	DINNER
MONDAY time			
TUESDAY time			
WEDNESDAY time			
THURSDAY time			
FRIDAY time			

trying them many times." Reluctantly Rebecca tasted a portion of spinach barely large enough to cover the tip of the fork.

"Gross-o!" screamed Rebecca.

"What do you mean, 'gross-o'?"

"This stuff stays in my mouth even after I swallow!"

A study by Herbert-Jackson et al. (1976) concluded that although familiarity with food may influence the food preferences of preschoolers to some extent, taste is the main influence.

Some of the foods that were most often rejected by the young children in this study come from the vegetable family. They are spinach, carrots, squash, broccoli, asparagus, okra, cauliflower, lima beans, and peas—vegetables with strong flavor.

The most preferred foods were from the meat group, all meats but liver. Favorites included chicken, hamburgers, hotdogs, and spaghetti with meat sauce.

The vegetables the children most preferred were corn, green beans, raw carrots, and mashed potatoes. The children seemed to be more or less indifferent to beets, green peppers, and most other vegetables. Noncitric fruits like apples, bananas, and grapes were the most preferred of the fruits.

Children's intake of fruits and vegetables is less varied than it should be. Their indifference to most dark green, leafy, and yellow vegetables means that many [approximately 66 percent according to a survey by Smiciklas-Wright et al. (1979)] consume inadequate amounts of vitamin C and food sources that provide vitamin A. Also limited in their diets, perhaps partly due to taste perferences and partly to a lack of familiarity with foods that provide them, are niacin, iron, and riboflavin.

Furthermore, a survey by Caliendo and Sanjur (1978) revealed that within a twenty-four-hour period, only 18 percent of the surveyed preschool population consumed adequate amounts of foods from each of the basic four food groups.

Implications for Menu Planning

It is, of course, wise to plan menus that reflect an awareness of the food preferences of young children. This, of course, saves money and promotes the child's feelings of security. But children should be exposed to and learn to eat a variety of foods. Those whose experience is limited to a few chosen foods will lack some of the essential nutrients needed for growth and the maintenance of health. It is, therefore, necessary to regularly include new and unfamiliar foods in the menu plan; to try to make "tasters" out of children. There are many ways to interest children in trying new foods. Involving children in menu planning and meal preparation are just two examples of techniques that work. Others are described in detail in Chapters 3, 4, 5, and 6.

Never offering a food is one way of prejudicing children toward it. To illustrate: In a report by Phillips and Kolasa (1980), children in Michigan child care centers were offered greens by only 4 percent of their parents and caregivers. Not surprisingly, over one-half of them classified greens as a vegetable most disliked, in addition to spinach and raw cauliflower. Preschoolers in the North Carolina centers, however, who also dislike spinach and raw cauliflower, listed greens, specifically collard greens, as a preferred food (Abdel-Ghany, 1978).

Because familiarity obviously plays such an important part in influencing food preference, adults who plan menus must try to find ways to expose young children to a variety of well-chosen foods. The most obvious, of course, is to include regularly new food items in the menu plans.

Menus for Children with Special Needs

In 1978 Public Law 94-142, the Education for All Handicapped Act was passed making it illegal to deny handicapped children between the ages of three and eighteen free, appropriate public education. As a result, many centers and schools have responded to parental requests to mainstream children with physical, emotional, and mental handicaps into their programs. These children frequently have limitations that affect the kind of foods they can eat and the ways in which they can be prepared and served. Moreover, because some medications deplete their systems of vital nutrients, their nutrient needs may also differ. The menu planners need to become familiar with their special needs by communicating closely and regularly with the parents.

Allergies are probably the most common problems children have that require modified diets. Since some allergic reactions can have serious consequences, it is necessary for caregivers and menu planners to keep an up-to-date list of all children and their food allergies posted in a highly visable place. Most often parents of these children will request written menus (which include snacks) in advance, so they can prepare substitute bag lunches on the days those foods are served.

Occasionally, parents will request that their children be served a vegetarian diet. The nutrient needs of these children will not be met if all meats and, in some cases, dairy products are removed from their plates, and they are merely given the vegetables and fruits that were planned for the other children's plates that day. You will need to combine vegetables and grains carefully to ensure the presence of all the essential amino acids required for proteins to be utilized by the body. A few combinations include *rice* with one of the following: wheat, sesame seeds, or legumes (soybeans, peanuts, black-eyed peas, kidney beans, chickpeas, navy beans, pinto beans, and lima beans). Other combinations are *legumes* (like those listed above) with either corn, rice, wheat, sesame seeds, barley, or oats; or *wheat* with legumes, soybeans and peanuts, soybeans and sesame seeds, or rice and soybeans.

Some families belong to religious orders that prohibit the consumption of certain foods. Jewish doctrine forbids the consumption of pork and shell fish; some Seventh Day Adventists practice vegetarian diets, and there are many other dietary restrictions imposed by other religious orders. Parents from these families may either pack their children's meals and snacks or ask that their child not be pressured to eat those foods which are objectionable to them if they are served. Of course, their wishes should be respected. Some schools and centers try hard to prepare foods that meet the needs of all of their children. Often this means adjusting the menu plan to accommodate these families.

MAINTAINING THE NUTRITIONAL INTEGRITY OF FOODS

Knowing how to plan menus to ensure an adequate nutrient balance assumes that when foods are bought and prepared they will contain the nutrients for which you chose them. Unfortunately, this is not always the case. Frequently, poorly handled foods, foods left in vegetable bins at the market for long periods of time, poorly refrigerated foods, foods frozen for too long, overcooked foods, and those left soaking in pots for hours all suffer a great loss of nutrients.

Nutrient loss begins from the time foods are harvested and continues until they reach the table. The degree of care taken to maintain their nutritional integrity will largly determine their nutritional value by the time they are consumed. A few pointers for conserving those nutrients are given below.

1. Buy fresh or frozen vegetables or fruit. If possible, grow some of your own. What a good experience gardening is for children! In addition to providing nutritious foods, the children would participate in a meaningful science experience.

2. When buying green leafy vegetables, look for those with the darkest leaves.

3. When buying yellow or orange vegetables, choose the darkest orange foods. Dark sweet potatoes contain more carotene (which provides vitamin A) than pale orange sweet potatoes, for example.

4. Don't allow foods to soak long before cooking. Soaking depletes water-soluble vitamins.

5. Cut fruits and vegetables that will be served raw just prior to serving them. Their vitamins are extremely perishable and quickly begin to dissipate when they are cut.

6. The practice of adding baking soda to beans destroys thiamin. Refrain from doing this.

7. Do not overcook vegetables. Cook them until they are just crunchy. The practice of letting vegetables, like green beans, stand in their pans while the older children are fed, and then pureeing them later for the infants is inappropriate. The beans should be cooked, pureed, and then quickly frozen to minimize nutrient loss.

8. Remember, the longer foods are left in the freezer, the more their nutrients dissipate.

9. Store canned foods in a cool place. Canned foods kept at above 80° F suffer a severe nutrient loss.

10. Wrap and refrigerate cooked or cut foods promptly.

11. Save vegetable and meat stocks for seasoning. Too often these nutrient-laden juices are poured down the sink. (Remove the fat from the meat stock, however.)

Serving Foods in a Sanitary Environment

Food, no matter how well prepared and presented, is only as good as it is clean and free from contamination. High standards of sanitation must be maintained in the purchase and preparation of foods to ensure healthful meals and snacks.

In many states, those who prepare and serve food in programs for young children are required to earn a food handler's certificate. Training for this certificate at least ensures that food handlers have a basic understanding of sanitary practices and that they are free from disease. In states where this certificate, or a comparable substitute, is not required, it is wise to consult the local department of health for information on sanitary food service practice. The meal management guides given at the end of this chapter can serve as additional references. Everyone who comes in contact with food must practice sanitary food management, even children.

Lee, a three-year-old, was overheard telling her friend not to eat an orange wedge, retrieved from the floor. "It has Germans on it," she said, adjusting the term "germs" to one with which she was familiar. Her friend examined the wedge closely, decided that no Germans were visible and, to Lee's dismay, promptly gobbled it up. Lee watched her friend closely to see what dreadful thing would happen as a result of eating the invisible "Germans."

Since bacteria are not visible, their threat is easy to overlook. Like Lee, though, we must maintain high standards of cleanliness when handling foods, aware that bacteria, though "invisible," are always present, and the potential for their growth in haphazard environments is great. High standards of sanitation must be maintained in the purchase, storage, service, and preparation of foods to ensure healthful meals and snacks.

Generally, there are three areas with which those who are responsible for creating and managing sanitary food program should be concerned. They are (1) personal hygiene and sanitary practices of food handlers, (2) controlling the growth and spread of food-borne bacteria, and (3) maintaining a clean and sterile setting in which to prepare and serve food. Each area is discussed below with a checklist of suggestions for promoting sanitary practice.

PERSONAL HYGIENE
AND SANITARY PRACTICE

Food service personnel and the children must maintain high standards of personal hygiene and sanitary practice. *The children should, for example,*

1. Learn to wash their hands thoroughly. Washing children's hands with a community cloth in a community bowl is unsanitary. Children can be encouraged to learn to wash their own hands by providing water play experiences. Follow this by putting a dab of a fragrant lotion on their hands and inviting them to enjoy the smooth, slippery feeling between their fingers and all over each part of their hands. Call attention to between the fingers and all areas of the palm.

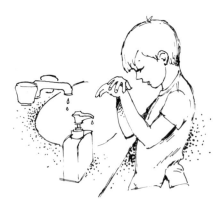

2. Be discouraged from eating left-over food from one another's plates and from passing food around.

3. Learn to swallow before talking to avoid spraying their neighbors with food.

The adults who prepare and serve food to children should

1. Wear clean clothes and have clean bodies.

2. Wear a hairnet or scarf if they work in the kitchen.

3. Wear no jewelry other than a watch or ring.

4. Wash hands and nails frequently, being careful not to recontaminate them by touching the faucet or basin when leaving. A clean paper towel should be used to dry hands, turn off the water, and to open the door to the lavatory.

5. If not well, refrain from handling food. If skin conditions exist, or if ill with a cold or the flu, it is unwise to handle food for others. One sneeze or cough can contaminate an entire work area, transmitting disease to other workers, children, and their families in a cycle that can last for months.

6. Taste foods from "tasting spoons" only. To taste, food should be transferred from a stirring spoon to the tasting spoon, which should then be placed immediately into the dishwashing area. The tasting spoon should never be returned to the food or be laid on the counter.

7. Wear plastic gloves whenever it is necessary to touch food with the fingers. Whenever possible, use tongs.

8. When serving or transporting containers of food or beverages, hold the container at the bottom. Do not let the thumbs hook over the rims and touch the contents of the bowls; likewise, the rims of cups which will come into contact with children's mouths.

BACTERIAL CONTAMINATION OF FOOD

Food-borne bacteria that can cause illness is frequently already present in food when it is purchased. Given moisture and a moderate temperature, these organisms can multiply rapidly. Some suggestions for controlling their growth and spreading are

1. Cook foods thoroughly. Salmonella cannot survive temperatures above 140° F.

2. Wash hands frequently and thoroughly during the cooking process. Staff and salmonella can spread via dirty hands, utensils, and equipment.

3. Do not use food from dented, bulging, or leaking cans. Likewise, canned foods that smell or look "offcolor" should be thrown out.

4. All foods should be thoroughly washed. This is particularly important for foods to be served raw.

5. Food should be stored in tightly covered containers in refrigerators and in cabinets and be labeled with the correct dates.

6. Use only pasteurized milk.

7. When buying food, inspect it carefully for container damage, spoilage, and cleanliness.

8. Keep food either *hot* (in excess of 140° F) or *cold* (below 40° F). Do not allow the food to cool to room temperature before placing it in the refrigerator. Instead, put it in shallow pans, and place the pans, unstacked, in the refrigerator. The center of the mass should cool to 45° F within 3 to 4 hours.

9. When heating foods, heat them in shallow dishes to ensure thorough heating throughout. This is especially important for casseroles and dishes with egg, tuna, and cream fillings.

MAINTAINING
A SANITARY FACILITY

The environment in which food is to be prepared and served must be kept clean and free of germs, insects, and rodents. Suggestions are as follows:

1. Examine food carefully for signs of insects or infestation. Be careful not to bring insects into the kitchen by way of food or grocery bags.

2. Be alert to signs of pest infestation, like insect or rodent droppings. If they are discovered, contact the health department for extermination advice.

3. Keep all work surfaces clean and free from clutter.

4. Wipe all cans before opening.

5. Scrub floors regularly with a disinfectant.

6. Wash dishes in detergent-slippery water heated to 110° to 120° F and rinse them by submerging whole racks in 120° to 140° F water for at least 30 seconds. A sanitizing agent such as clorine should be added to the water.

7. Scrub the refrigerator frequently. Do not line it, as this prevents air from circulating to cool foods rapidly.

For those who wish additional guidance in menu planning or evaluating their food service operation, state health departments, home extension services, welfare departments, hospital dietary departments, WIC centers, the Child Care Food Program sponsored by the U.S. Department of Agriculture, or Head Start Centers employ professional dietitians and nutritionists who can serve as consultants to your programs. They can help to plan or evaluate a series of menus or provide training for your food service personnel. The service of foods, nutrition, and the social and psychological aspects of eating are areas in which they are particularly helpful.

REVIEW ACTIVITIES

1. Visit the local welfare department and ask to speak to the licensing specialist for child care centers. Find out what certification or training is required for those who wish to prepare and serve food to children.
2. Call the local health department. Find out the procedure and schedule for inspecting kitchens in child care centers and what standards must be maintained.

3. Contact a WIC center or a home extension agent, and find out what it would cost to hire someone to
   a. Plan a monthly series of nutritionally balanced menus that include lunches and snacks.
   b. Evaluate a cycle of menus that you have already planned and make recommendations for improvement.
   c. Provide a nutrition in-service training session for caregivers or parents.
4. Review three books on food service and sanitary food practice.
5. Visit a child care center during lunch time and
   a. Evaluate the menu based on the checklist provided in this chapter. List each food item. Rate each (1 to 3) according to children's response to them. For example, 1 = "all gone"; 2 = tasted; 3 = left mostly untouched.
   b. How do your findings compare with the discussion of food preferences given in this chapter?

SUGGESTED READINGS

ADAMS, C.F., *Nutritive Values of American Foods in Common Units*, Agriculture Handbook, no. 456, Agricultural Research Service, U.S. Department of Agriculture. Washington, D.C.: U.S. Government Printing Office, 1975.

FONOSCH, G., and KVITKA, E.F., *Meal Management*. New York: Canfield Press, 1978.

KINDER, F., and GREEN, N.R., *Meal Management*. New York: MacMillan, Inc., 1978.

SMICIKLAS-WRIGHT, HELEN, and FLORENCE PETERSEN, and DONALD PETERS, "Day Care Nutrition Programs and Children's Home Diets," *Child Care Quarterly*, Spring 1979, pp. 47-58.

U.S. Department of Agriculture (Food and Nutrition Service), *Child Care Food Program*, FNS-154m. Washington, D.C.: U.S. Department of Agriculture, 1976.

_____, *Quantity Recipes for Child Care Centers*, FNS-86. Washington, D.C.: U.S. Department of Agriculture, May 1973.

U.S. Office of the Federal Register, "School Lunch Requirements," *Federal Register* 42:175. Washington, D.C.: U.S. Government Printing Office, 1975.

chapter two

feeding **INFANTS**
and **TODDLERS**

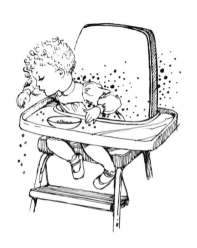

OBJECTIVES

After reading this chapter the reader will be able to:

- Describe some of the physical needs and psychological demands of infants and toddlers during feeding time.
- Discuss the importance of snacks in the toddler's daily menu plan.

Eleven-month-old Tracy leaned forward, straining to watch the peas as she dropped them, one by one, over the edge of her feeding tray and onto the floor. When they were "all gone," she squealed and banged on her tray for more, which she promptly began dropping faster and more gleefully than ever.

Tracy's newfound ability to release, at will, an object from between her index finger and thumb was an exciting discovery that took precedence over her hunger. The peas and the highchair provided the perfect opportunity to practice this new skill.

The eating behavior of infants and toddlers is frequently messy and frustrating to adults. However, Tracy's behavior is appropriate for her developmental level. As toddlers strive to master their environments, all available materials are fair game for sensorial exploration! Tasting an occasional pea was only incidental as she enthusiastically practiced finger-thumb independence and explored physical laws, noting how objects of different sizes, shapes, and weights move through space and over surfaces.

The messiness of infants and toddlers during mealtime makes coping with exuberant exploratory behavior difficult for adults who are pressed for time and patience. The way in which adults respond to the eating behavior of young children, however, can facilitate growth or result in mealtimes filled with tantrums and sulky manipulating behaviors. Patience, skill, and an understanding of the developmental needs of children at each stage are required if positive eating habits are to be promoted.

The psychological and physical factors that influence eating behavior in infants and toddlers are many and may be as important as are the choices that adults make regarding what children are to be fed and when. In this chapter, some of those factors are examined and practical suggestions given.

FEEDING INFANTS

When caring for an infant, much of the time during the day must be devoted to preparing food, feeding, cleaning, and diapering. For that reason, the adult-child ratio for infants in group care should be low: one adult for every three infants is a suggested ratio.

As any mother of twins can testify, even the task of feeding two hungry infants is a challenge! In group care, the crying of one hungry infant often stimulates neighboring infants to cry. Sometimes it is difficult to determine which infant is crying from hunger and who is merely joining the chorus!

Individual variations in feeding schedules, behavior, and elimination schedules can be more readily learned if each caregiver is responsible for the primary care of the same infants each day. Not only will the caregiver become sensitized to individual behaviors that signal hunger or discomfort, but this practice also helps to promote attachments which are necessary for optimum social and emotional development.

When, and How Much?

Because the growth rates and activity levels of infants differ, their feeding requirements and habits likewise differ. It is important for adults to be sensitive to and tolerant of these individual variations. Often adjustments in feeding schedules and serving sizes must be made to accommodate the changing needs of the growing infant if a secure emotional environment is to be provided.

Because babies have small stomachs, they will need to eat more frequently than older children. Their behavior is the best indicator of their needs; when they are hungry, they will signal a desire to be fed, usually by crying. Since crying is one of a baby's few means of controlling the environment insensitive or unresponsive adults who ignore the baby's cues will frustrate the infant's emerging sense of competency and trust.

Babies signal satiation by turning away from food or by becoming easily distracted from eating. This behavior should cue the adult to discontinue feeding. Trying to tease the infant to nurse longer or to consume more is a form of forced feeding that can contribute to obesity and that is not conducive to learning to eat in moderation. Likewise, adding cereal to the bottle in an effort to extend the period of time between feedings is not a sound practice. Animal studies suggest that small, frequent feedings are more likely to promote good health than less frequent, larger meals. Trying to extend the periods between feedings by stuffing the infants with cereal or forcing the last drop from the bottle seems to be a practice that exists mainly for the convenience of adults. Given time, the infant will grow and become able to comfortably accommodate larger quantities of milk and other solid foods. Until then, young infants may signal to be fed *every* two or three hours. Some pediatricians, however, perhaps in response to parent pressure will arbitrarily set a four-hour interval feeding schedule.

The nutritional requirements of most healthy infants will be met by consuming approximately 2 to 3 ounces per pound of body weight of formula containing 20 kilocalories per ounce during a twenty-four-hour period. A record of the daily intake should be kept and made available to parents when they arrive to take the infant home. Likewise, changes in elimination habits should be recorded and presented to parents regularly.

Feeding Infants in a Group Setting

For the first six months of life, milk is the primary source of food for humans. The mothers of some infants will wish for them to have breast milk even though the demands of their jobs may absent them from the nursing scene. Other infants will be provided with formula, especially prepared and labeled for them. In both cases, the wishes of the parent should be respected.

Breast-Fed Infants

It is generally thought that breast-feeding provides optimal sanitary conditions and a perfect balance of the nutrients that are necessary for normal growth. It is the method recommended by the American Academy of Pediatrics. Some doctors will, however, recommend vitamin, fluoride, and iron supplements for breast-fed infants.

Working mothers can prepare the milk for the day's feeding in advance by expressing it painlessly from one breast while the infant is nursing the other. The milk should be poured from the expression cup into a plastic bottle liner, secured at the top and labeled with the date and names of the infant and the caregiving adult. Several liners may be placed inside a larger freezer bag and may be frozen. The breast milk may remain frozen for up to six days before deterioration begins. When needed, the milk should be thawed out in the refrigerator, not in a warm room. The liner can then be placed in a plastic form, capped with a sterilized nipple, and offered to the infant. Ideally, it should be tasted to check for freshness before it is given to the infant (breast milk is very sweet and has a white, watery consistency). Some parents prefer that the bottle be warmed to room temperature before it is offered to the infant.

Formula Feeding

Normal development can be achieved with formula feeding also. The choice of formula should be the joint responsibility of the parent and pediatrician. Once selected, it should not be altered in any way by the caregiver. The practice of adding syrup or cereal to formulas is unacceptable. If a caregiver feels that the formula is inadequate or that it fails to provide for the nutrient needs of the infant, careful notes describing the baby's behavior, intake, sleeping patterns, and elimination should be recorded at regular intervals during the day. These findings should be presented to the parent. The baby's parent, after conferring with a doctor, may then decide to alter the formula.

Currently, a great deal of information regarding the care and feeding of infants exists; much of it is conflicting and confusing to parents. Caregivers should try to avoid becoming another source of undue frustration or alarm for the family. Therefore, concerns relating to the baby's feeding should be communicated with care and sensitivity, and only after careful documentation of specific events that may signal a problem. For example, gross deviations from normal weight may indicate the need for nutrition counseling. If the infant frequently vomits, has diarrhea, or shows a general lack of interest in feeding, this behavior must also be reported to the parent with as much specificity as possible. Such behavior could signal the onset of allergies or lactose intolerance, a condition most prevalent in premature infants and black and oriental children. Both conditions often require that an infant's formula be changed, but a physician's advice should first be sought by the parent. Since the physician will need to know of the specific events of symptoms that have given rise to concern, the information provided by the caregiver becomes a valuable tool to aid in diagnosing illness.

Formula Preparation

When preparing a formula, the directions of the manufacturer must be closely followed. Concentrated formulas must be carefully diluted to prevent constipation. Watering down the formula, however, will produce nutrient deficiencies and eventual starvation. Ideally, the formula should be prepared on site by the caregiver to ensure freshness and sanitation. In some states, this is a requirement.

Sanitary conditions must prevail if infections from the use of unclean bottles, nipples, can openers, funnels, and spoons are to be prevented. Bottles should be used only once before they are resterilized, and hands should be washed before touching any of the feeding paraphernalia, whether to clean it or to present it to the baby. To avoid mix-ups, milk should be labeled with the date and each child's name before it is stored in the refrigerator to await its use.

The Nursling

A new infant's eyes can focus on an object no further away than 9 inches. Interestingly, that is the approximate distance between the breast and the adult face! The infant who is cuddled during feeding time is not only provided with physical nourishment, but nuturance, which promotes trust, attachment, security, and opportunities to develop newly emerging visual skills.

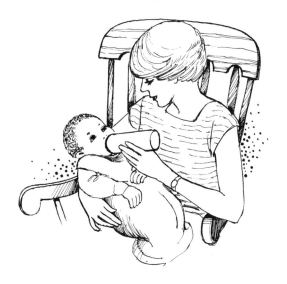

The practice of bottle propping, on the other hand, deprives the infant of these important experiences and may also promote ear infections and dental caries. When an infant falls asleep in the crib while nursing, milk can dribble down and enter the ear, providing a ripe medium for bacterial growth, which can cause ear infections. Moreover, the milk sugars left in the mouth coat the gums and, if left undisturbed, slowly invade the newly crowning teeth, causing caries, a condition frequently referred to as "nursing-bottle syndrome." Ideally, a baby's new teeth should be wiped with a sterile cloth or soft towel following each feeding.

Before feeding the baby, place a bib under the chin and find a relatively quiet place to sit with the infant cuddled closely in a semisitting position. Hold the bottle so that the nipple is always filled with milk. The nipple may need to be adjusted to provide just the right rate of flow for the baby.

When the baby appears to be satiated, perhaps showing you by blowing bubbles or letting milk run freely from the sides of its mouth, it is time to stop feeding. Hold the infant upright for at least fifteen minutes to prevent regurgitation. The baby will also need a gentle massage or a little back patting to bring up a burp once or twice during and following the feeding. When the infant is placed in the crib for a nap following a feeding, it is best to prop the baby on its right side to prevent aspiration of regurgitated milk.

Introducing
Solid Foods to Infants

Controversy abounds regarding the optimum age for introducing solid foods to infants. Most doctors agree that infants should be offered sterile water at about two weeks after birth, since pound for pound, their water requirements exceed that of adults. The age for introducing solid foods, however, remains the subject of vigorous discussion.

Some parents are encouraged, largely by friends and relatives, to introduce cereal to the diet of their infants as early as two months of age; others are advised to wait a full year. The American Academy of Pediatrics, however, recommends giving the infant solid food between four and six months, the age at which an infant is able to sit with support and has already developed the required neuromuscular control for manipulating food and swallowing. At this age, the infant can indicate an interest in eating by leaning forward or satiation by turning away. Introducing solids before this level of development is reached may interfere with the establishment of sound eating habits, aggravate food allergies, and contribute to obesity.

Baby's First Foods

Iron-fortified rice, oat, or barley cereals are generally the first foods offered to infants, since these grains are less likely to provoke allergies. The first feeding should consist of approximately 1 teaspoon of cereal, thinly mixed with a few tablespoons of lukewarm formula or breast milk. The amount should be gradually increased and offered to the infant daily for the first eighteen months of life.

Surprising things happen when an infant experiences the new taste, texture, and consistency of cereal! Much of it—perhaps most of it—will dribble from the corners of the infant's mouth; the remainder may be pushed out with the tongue. This doesn't mean that the baby doesn't like cereal, just that it takes time for the infant to acquire the skills required to manipulate solid food to the back of the mouth and to swallow. With a small, shallow spoon, place the cereal near the back of the baby's tongue and continue to scoop it back into the baby's mouth while the baby "practices" this important skill.

It is important to allow time for the baby to get used to the cereal; wait at least a week before introducing another solid food. In the meantime, watch the infant for signs of an allergic reaction (coughing, vomiting, or rashes). If the baby seems to thrive on this new diet, it is time to consider adding additional solids, again at the rate of one new food per week.

Either commercially prepared or home-prepared foods may be chosen for the next addition to the diet. In most cases this decision is made by the parent and doctor. If the infant is cared for in a center, however, state regulations regarding food service for infants and children in group settings may prohibit the parent from sending in food. The food for the infant, in this case, would be prepared or purchased by the center.

Commercially Prepared Foods

If center policy mandates or parent requests dictate commercially prepared foods for the next addition to the baby's diet, they should be selected with care, since the amount of calories and essential nutrients in commercial preparations varies. Important information regarding the nutritional value of each infant food is printed on the label and should be carefully studied to ensure an adequate selection.

At each feeding, enough food, beginning with ½ teaspoon and gradually increasing to a maximum of 1 tablespoon, should be removed from the jar and served to the infant from a sterile bowl or plate. Serving directly from the jar allows bacteria to build up in the left-over portions and, therefore, should be avoided. All food from opened jars should be covered, dated, and refrigerated. Uneaten portions should be discarded after forty-eight hours.

Fruits and Vegetables Prepared "from Scratch"

Foods prepared "from scratch" should be either fresh or frozen. Food that is marketed in cans, not especially prepared for infants, frequently contains high levels of sodium, sugar, and sometimes lead. Since we know relatively little about the effects of early imprinting on food preferences, it is perhaps better to avoid feeding infants most salted, canned vegetables and fruits packed in heavy syrup. Moreover, additional salt and sweeteners should not be added to their foods.

It is also important to avoid overcooking food in order to minimize oxidation of vitamins and to blend or puree foods only slightly before straining them in order to maintain their nutritional integrity. Once prepared, several servings can be frozen in cubes for up to a month. Food that is refrigerated, but not frozen, must be served or discarded within twenty-four hours.

Which Comes First, Fruits or Vegetables?

General disagreement exists over the question of whether fruits or vegetables should be the first food to be served to infants following the introduction of cereals. Many adults fear that if the infant first develops a preference for fruits, which are naturally sweet, vegetables may be rejected when they are offered later. Research suggests that infants inately prefer sweets, if given a choice. For this reason, the somewhat time-honored practice of introducing vegetables first seems a reasonable practice. On the other hand, if fruits are offered first, vegetables can be introduced by combining them with a fruit that has already found favor with the infant.

Regardless of which food is offered first, vegetables or fruits should be given in small amounts (approximately ½ teaspoon the first day, increasing to a maximum amount of 1 tablespoon per serving per year of life) one at a time, with careful monitoring of the infant's physical and emotional responses to each food. Waiting a week before adding a new food allows the caregiver to pinpoint responses that may signal an allergic reaction. Negative reactions may indicate a need to postpone adding some foods to the diet.

When fruits and vegetables are well established in the diet, meats and egg yolks may be offered. Some adults find the smell, texture, and flavor of pureed meats to be offensive. Infants, who are sensitive to nonverbal cues, also become prejudiced to them when adults hold their noses, shudder, or gag while serving pureed meats. Having no previous experience with grilled steaks and lamb chops, infants have no basis for comparisons and will, no doubt, find strained meats to be more interesting if they are served with enthusiasm.

As infants grow in their ability to tolerate many new foods, some of their pureed foods can be replaced with well-cooked finger foods.

Self-Feeding Skills

Babies love to help feed themselves! They will show you by putting their hands in their mouths while their mouths are full and by grabbing the spoon and refusing to let go. By the end of a feeding session, their food is likely to cover the feeding tray, floor, their hair, and you. Adults who are bothered by this messy, exuberant style of skill practice will need to reevaluate their expectations. Restrictions and unreasonable demands for neatness will create tensions and impede normal progress in the development of this new skill.

It takes a lot of practice to learn to pickup just the right amount of food, bring it to the mouth, and put it in, unaided. For that reason, it is a good idea to include some finger foods in the beginning; peas, cooked carrots, and small pieces of diced potatoes are examples of foods with which infants can practice independent eating skills.

To reduce the baby's urge to grab the spoon as you try to aim it quickly for its mouth, place a spoon in the baby's other hand. The baby can use that one for waving and banging. When you think the child is ready, place some mashed potatoes or other sticky food on the spoon, and let the child try to lick it off. With delighted encouragement from the caregiver, the infant will soon be fairly independent at mealtime.

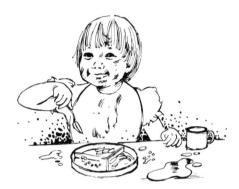

Food Pacifiers

Food should not be used as a pacifier, no matter how well it serves to keep babies quiet and occupied! Hard breads like zwieback or enriched baby cookies, which are frequently used to soothe teething babies, should be limited to no more than three or four a day, even if they are enriched.

The bottle is also an inappropriate pacifier. Moreover, the Academy of Pediatrics recommends that bottle feedings be limited to milk and water. Other beverages, including orange juice, should be served in a cup when the child is mature enough to drink from one. Since orange juice is particularly difficult for many infants to digest, many pediatricians recommend withholding it until the child is about a year old.

Food Preferences of Infants

From the beginning, some infants will indicate strong preferences for certain foods and will reject others outright. Food that is rejected should be offered again later, when the baby is really hungry, perhaps by combining it with a favorite food. It is important to use this early exploratory period to introduce the infant to a variety of tastes and not to allow the infant to settle for a few favorites. Infants whose diets include a wide range of foods will most likely achieve a balance of all the nutrients needed for their rapidly growing bodies.

TODDLERS, GROWING LESS AND EATING LESS

Infants normally double their weight by their first birthday; a one-year-old girl will weigh about 18 to 23 pounds. One can imagine the result if toddlers continued to grow at this rate—doubling their weight every year. A five-year-old could weigh a whopping 320 pounds!

During the second year of life, toddlers experience a vastly decelerated rate of weight gain, gaining only 4 to 5 pounds. This diminished rate of gain results in a reduced appetite, an occurrence that frequently triggers alarm in adults who worry that the toddler may not be getting the nourishment needed for growth. Moreover, the appetites of toddlers come and go rather unpredictably. It is not unusual, for example, for two-year-olds to eat very little for two days and then to gorge on the third day. Adults should take comfort in remembering that healthy toddlers will eat when their bodies need food. Therefore, food that is offered to them at these important times should be of superior nutritional quality.

Breakfast is the meal that is most often eaten with gusto. Normally finicky toddlers seem to have a bottomless pit between 6:00 and 8:30 A.M., and they seem to enjoy breakfast more than any other meal.

Breakfast is the meal that literally fuels the body and brain for the day's activities. The body, although in a state of rest for approximately ten hours during the night, continues to grow, and the calories that are used for this growth must be replaced. Therefore, a good breakfast with an ample protein food (meat, peanut butter, eggs) should be offered to the toddler. Also, a fruit, whole-grain or enriched bread, and/or cereal and milk or a milk product should be included. Some breakfast favorites for toddlers are as follows:

- *Cheesetoast* or grilled cheese
- *Apple wedges* with peanut butter spread
- *Left-over supper meats,* like chicken slices
- *Hard-boiled eggs,* which the toddler can peel independently
- *Pancakes* rolled into blankets for cottage cheese, fruit, or meat surprises
- *Hot cereals* with raisins, cream, and fruit
- *Raw vegetable slices* with a hard-boiled egg and a nutritious dip
- *Fruit kabobs,* alternating fruits on party toothpicks (adult supervision is required to ensure that the toothpicks are handled carefully.)
- *Cereals,* dry, whole-grain, and unsweetened

Unlike other meals during which toddlers often seem distractible and fidgety, breakfast can be enjoyed in relative peace and serve to tame the toddler for a good morning start. Sometimes the toddler's early morning misbehavior and short-temper can be attributed to a nutritionally inferior breakfast or to not being fed at all.

FEEDING TODDLERS

Occasionally at mealtimes, the toddler will issue a balky "no!" when prodded to eat. This behavior signals the first real visible evidence of the toddler's drive for autonomy. If adults ignore these important "no's" and continue to try to bribe and force them to eat more, eating behavior can become a tool for manipulating and controlling adults, often provoking thrilling outbursts of anger and frustration from adults.

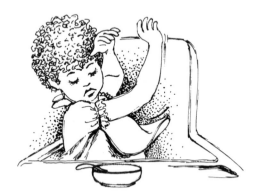

If, however, the adult recognizes the child's diminished appetite as a natural physical response to a slower rate of growth, peace may once again be restored. Even the most perceptive adult, however, may sometimes be confounded by a toddler's behavior at mealtime, as evidenced by the following episode.

"Eat your ice cream before it melts, Hank," the caregiver prodded.
"No."
"But it's your favorite kind. It has strawberries in it."

"I don't want it." The caregiver sighed as he removed it from the table and began to clear the dishes. Hank sank down into the chair and began to sniffle, and then to whine. "What's the matter now, Hank?" the caregiver asked.

"I want my ice cream," cried Hank, as tears of disappointment came streaming down his cheeks.

Often in their bid for autonomy, toddlers refuse those things that are most wanted by them. This behavior appears to be a kind of test, to determine if anyone will listen to them or respect their wishes. The wise adult will be sensitive to the child's need to gain control over their environment and the events that affect them. This is sometimes a painful process for adults and children alike. In this case, the loss of a perishable item as a natural consequence of refusing the ice cream provided a meaningful lesson for Hank.

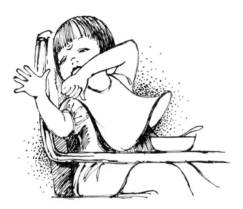

Food Jags

Another source of mealtime contention are the food jags of toddlers, as predictable in a toddler as crying is for infants. Two- and three-year-olds will often eat only one food to the exclusion of others for a period of time. The demand for hotdogs, for example, may be preempted the next week by a demand for spaghetti. These food jags are not harmful, as long as nutritious snacks are provided throughout the day to balance the diet. Food jags that extend beyond a few weeks, however, may be a cause for concern. Most food jags last only a week or so at a time.

Snacktime for Toddlers

Most toddlers have difficulty sitting for long periods of time and are frequently less interested in the mealtime experience than adults would like them to be. Because of toddlers' inability to sit still for long periods and because of their relatively small intake capacity, snacks provide an important addition to their daily diet. Left on their own, they will not choose foods that are best for them. Therefore, snacks should be chosen by the adult to provide a balance in the daily menu plan.

Nutritious snacks can be made available in small portions at any time in the morning or afternoon, until about 90 minutes before mealtime. Most toddlers will wish to carry snacks around the room with them as they play or investigate the activities of their friends. It is probably a better idea, however, to require them to sit wherever the snack is served and perhaps listen to a record or chat with a friend until they have finished.

This is an exciting time for making new food discoveries. Two-year-olds are most often inquisitive and ready to try out new foods at snacktime. Three-year-olds, however, are a little more cautious. According to Birch (1979), three-year-olds most readily accept only foods they can identify; they are highly suspicious of unfamiliar foods. It is important, therefore, for snacks not to be thrust upon children with little regard for their need to approach the new foods cautiously. To prod them may begin a whole cycle of feeding problems. Snacks should be offered in creative and appetizing ways, some of which are described in Chapters 4, 5, and 6.

Some easy-to-handle, popular finger snacks for children "on the go" are carrots, apple wedges, crackers with spreads, finger sandwiches, wieners, and rolled meats.

Encouraging the Assertive Behavior of Toddlers at Mealtime

Most toddlers graduate entirely from "junior foods" to table foods by two years of age. Physically, they will have developed teeth required for chewing fibrous foods, and emotionally, they will have matured enough to make their preferences and needs readily known. They will not only demand to feed themselves, but they should be encouraged to do so. This proves, however, to be a messy venture!

It is necessary to provide an adequate and supportive environment to accompany this assertive behavior. At mealtime, a very large bib; child-sized furniture and utensils that are unbreakable, untippable, and easy for unpracticed hands to manage; and, if the floor cannot be mopped, a plastic floor covering, perhaps a shower curtain, are a few of the supplies needed to provide a safe, worry-free setting. Here are additional tips for encouraging initiative in toddlers and for ensuring a pleasant mealtime experience.

1. Hands should be washed by the toddler in a sink with running water. The practice of using the same cloth and water for all of the children should be discouraged.

2. Allow the children to help set the table. Begin by placing a plate at each place. Ask toddler helpers to put a napkin at each setting. Other helpers can distribute cups, spoons, and/or forks, and put a bib on each chair.

3. Place one or two small durable plastic pitchers of milk on each table. The pitchers should have easy-grip handles and dripless spouts. Yes, toddlers can pour their own milk to a premarked line on their cups (about one-

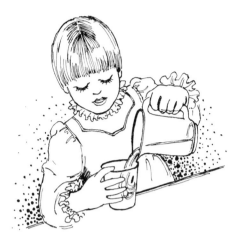

half full). Children who have difficulty pouring will need additional water-play experiences and opportunities to practice pouring in sand, rice, or water tables.

4. Cloth bibs with velcro fasteners can be fastened by the children, thus promoting independence and the development of initiative. Occasionally, in the beginning, they may need to ask a friend to help them. When bibs are removed, they can be rinsed, used to wipe the toddler's face, and then thrown into the laundry basket.

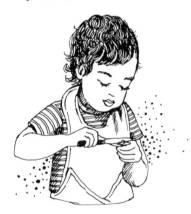

5. If desserts are served, serve them with the meal to avoid being tempted to use the dessert for a bribe. If they are "nutrient dense," they can be an important addition to the meal. Desserts like fruits, custards, or yogurt topped with wheat germ are examples of appropriate desserts.

6. Mealtime is not a time for power struggles. Postpone disputes; resolve them later, after the meal. Toddlers become frustrated easily and, when pressured to conform to adult standards, they may rebel. For this reason, the adult should eliminate the factors in the emotional and physical environment that can cause undue stress at mealtime.

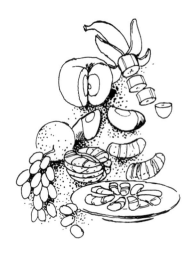

7. Remember that refined table manners emerge slowly during the maturing process. Be a model for good manners, displaying an appreciative attitude toward the food that is served.

8. Refrain from prodding or forcing children to clean their plates. Keep serving sizes small with options for second helpings. One tablespoon from each of the food groups for each year of life is a suggested guideline. Remember, children will eat when they are hungry. Some children because of different energy requirements will need more; others will need less.

9. Be tolerant when toddlers experiment with their foods. They will examine each new offering closely. Squishing, smearing, and sometimes blowing bubbles is a part of the exciting process of learning about foods.

CONCLUSION

It is important for adults to be concerned, not only with the physical demands of feeding, but also with the psychological needs of infants and young children during feeding time. The nurturance given and the adult's attention and sensitivity to the emotional needs of the infant during feeding are perhaps as important as the need to clean bottles, nipples, and caps. Nurturing involves touching, holding, and interacting, and feeding time provides optimal opportunities for nurturing play.

Toddlers, although not as fragile as infants, have nutritional needs that are as demanding. A creative and patient approach is required to interest the two- or three-year-old in trying new foods and developing positive dietary habits during snack and mealtimes.

Nutritious snacks—an important part of the toddler's daily nutrient intake—help to replenish the energy spent in play and provide the nutrients required for growth. Therefore, snacks should be chosen with care from the basic four food groups and offered in supportive surroundings that encourage the newly emerging assertive behavior of toddlers.

Infants and toddlers who are given an opportunity to develop a taste for a variety of new foods during this early period of exploration and discovery will have taken the first, important steps toward developing sound eating habits that can last a lifetime.

REVIEW ACTIVITIES

1. Visit a center that provides care for infants and toddlers during lunchtime. Describe the procedures for feeding
   a. Infants
      (1) Are infants fed on demand?
      (2) How are feedings scheduled?
      (3) Are infants held during feeding time?
      (4) How does the center provide for breast-fed babies?
      (5) Are the babies' intakes recorded?
      (6) Are they reported to parents? How?
      (7) Who determines what babies are to be fed?
   b. Toddlers
      (1) Describe the meal and how the children responded to each item.
      (2) Were the adults seated and interacting with the toddlers, or did they hover above them?
      (3) How was responsibility and independence encouraged by the physical setting and adult responses?
      (4) What special utensils, bibs, and chairs were used?
      (5) What provisions for handwashing were made prior to mealtime?
      (6) Can you think of any suggestions that could have been followed to improve the mealtime atmosphere?
2. Survey at least five young parents. Ask them to describe the nutrition counseling they have received from friends, relatives, and their child's physician. What were they told regarding
   a. Which to serve first—fruits or vegetables?
   b. How to get the baby to sleep through the night?
   c. Whether or not the child needs a nutrient supplement?
   d. How to determine an appropriate serving size?
3. Visit a pediatrician's office. If possible, get copies of the nutrition information they pass along to new parents.

chapter three

feeding
PRESCHOOL
children

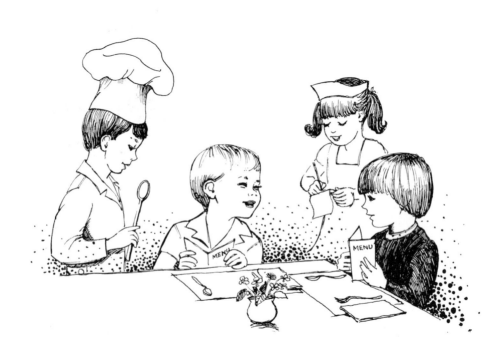

OBJECTIVES

After reading this chapter the reader will be able to:

- Create a mealtime setting that promotes good eating habits.
- Develop strategies for influencing the food preferences and overcoming the food prejudices of preschool children.
- Serve meals in a variety of creative ways.

The atmosphere of discovery and exploration that prevails in most child care settings and schools provides an ideal climate for developing positive dietary habits and attitudes in young children. Curiosity about unfamiliar foods is piqued when children observe their peers enjoying new foods. Even appreciation for familiar foods is enhanced when children see adults other than their relatives eating and enjoying foods that may have previously seemed uninteresting to them. Lunch and snacktime in such a setting offer vast opportunities for social interaction and the achievement of nutritional goals.

Just as the nutrient requirements and food intake patterns of four- and five-year-olds differ considerably from those of infants and toddlers (see Table 1-2), so do some of the methods that should be used by adults to promote positive dietary habits in preschoolers. How children are fed greatly influences what they will eat. Therefore, this chapter presents ways to create an environment that promotes good dietary habits in young children. Presented are some practical methods for overcoming food prejudices, techniques for introducing new foods, some common adult behaviors that impede the development of good dietary habits in young children, and some creative ideas for varying dull mealtime routines.

BREAKFAST AND SNACKTIME

Children most often arrive at different times in the morning. Some have eaten a healthful breakfast; others have been rushed out, given little or nothing to eat. Many parents believe their children are fed at school or the center; they may count on it. If the center does not provide the parent with a regular menu plan for each day, the parent is likely to rely on their children to tell them whether or not they were served breakfast. And since children are likely to confuse snack and breakfast times, the information they give their parents may not be reliable.

Children who are not given breakfast at home or at the caregiver's have a long time to wait between suppertime and their midmorning snack the next day! If that snack consists of only cookies and a fruit drink, children may become irritable and their behavior unmanageable before lunchtime.

Since hungry children are frequently unable to cope with the normal challenges of the morning's activities, a cooking activity the first thing in the morning or a self-serve snack table made available to all the children may provide the solution. The cooking activity could allow for some "munching" as the food is prepared. Or, if a self-serve snack table is used, some foods should be served that can be managed independently by the children, such as preportioned or precut fruits, vegetables, or meats; milk or juice in child-sized pitchers; unsweetened cereals; hard-cooked eggs; and whole-wheat muffins or breads with various spreads.

Later in the morning, about 90 minutes before the noon meal, a small snack coordinated with the menu plan for the day should be served to all the children. Some suggestions for snacks that can be prepared by the children with minimum adult supervision are as follows (other snacktime ideas and recipes can be found in Chapters 4 and 5):

- *Popcorn*—Substitute grated parmesan cheese for butter and salt
- *Omelets* with "choose your own" fillings
- *Potatoes,* mashed, with cheese
- *Potato pancakes and waffles* with applesauce and other fruit toppings, nuts, granola, peanut butter, or cottage cheese
- *French toast* with whole-wheat bread and no additional sugar in the batter.
- *Orange juice,* freshly squeezed. It is important to remember that "fruit drinks" are not fruit *juices.* Even those fruit punches that have been fortified with vitamins often lack important vitamins and minerals and contain high levels of sugar and salt.
- *Shakes* made by mixing juices with milk and ice
- *Baked apples* with raisins, nuts, or spices
- *Yogurt* with fruit, granola, or nuts
- *Hot cereals* with yogurt, raisins, or ice cream
- *Dates* or *Apricots* stuffed with peanut butter
- *Cooked pumpkin* with butter and spices
- *Eggs,* poached, with cheese
- *Cottage cheese* mixed with fresh fruit, applesauce, sesame seeds, wheat germ, or granola
- *Whole-wheat toast* with peanut butter

While snacks and self-serve breakfasts can be served informally, lunchtime is most often a sit-down affair and requires effort and planning to provide an optimal nutritional environment.

The U.S. Department of Agriculture Child Nutrition Program mandates that all children who are served in group programs receiving USDA funds must be provided with no less than one-third of their RDA at lunchtime. Therefore, those who prepare this important meal must not only be aware of the nutritional requirements of young children but know how to serve food in ways that will appeal to children. Food not eaten because of a tense, poorly planned mealtime setting will not provide any nutrients.

Providing a Supportive Physical and Emotional Setting at Mealtime

The physical and emotional climate in which meals are served has an important impact on the appetites of young children. Children, like adults, are likely to respond with a loss of appetite to a mealtime sprinkled with generous portions of bribery, ultimatums, and threats. By evaluating the emotional and physical setting and anticipating problems that are likely to occur due to poor planning, the potential for mishaps and negative exchanges between adults and children can be minimized.

Begin by providing the children with chairs and tables that "fit the children." They cannot be expected to sit properly at the table if their feet don't touch the floor. Moreover, the table should be low enough to allow the children to manipulate their flatware comfortably and to elevate their noses up

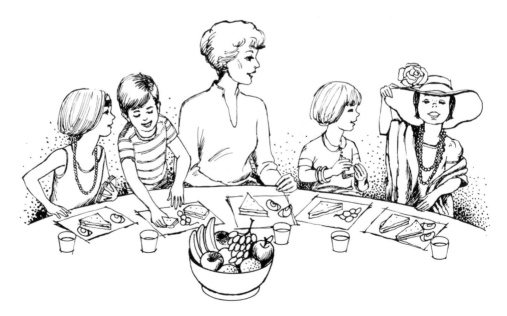

and away from steamy vegetables that can be disagreeable when in close proximity to one's nose.

A family-style seating arrangement is preferable to long benches and tables for small children. Four to six children at a table with one adult who rotates from table to table daily or weekly is ideal. This system provides the adult with an opportunity to observe the eating habits of individual children, to draw them into conversation, and to model appropriate eating habits and manners for them. It is not a good time to "train" children by calling attention to inappropriate behavior or mistakes. These should be noted, however, and used as a plan for teaching, perhaps through role play at a later time. Attention should not be focused on a child who is reluctant to eat. This merely reinforces noneating behavior. It is more helpful for the adult to model positive eating habits, perhaps by commenting on the positive habits of other children under supervision. Moreover, it is especially important that the adult eat whatever the children are served and with gusto!

The seating arrangements may be formal or informal. Children may be allowed to choose where they wish to be seated, or they may be assigned seats. Some children seem to feel more secure if they are allowed to eat at the same place every day. Others seem to enjoy choosing their own place or sitting beside different children each day. A compromise can be accomplished for the child who needs a "sense of place" by using name cards at the table. Children who cannot read print can "read" picture stickers if they are attached to the cards beside the child's name. Place cards can be kept at the same place for the comfort of the more cautious child and rotated for or by the other children who wish to choose their own spaces.

Flexible seating arrangements allow for changes to be made in response to individual needs. For example, it may occasionally be advantageous to seat a finicky eater beside a child who relishes a variety of foods. In this way, modeling can be used to expand a scanty diet.

Tables can be set by a team of children before the meal. Children can be assigned table setting tasks on a rotating basis by using a chart with their names and symbols that stand for each task on it. Try to program each job for success. For example, place mats with silouettes of the utensils drawn

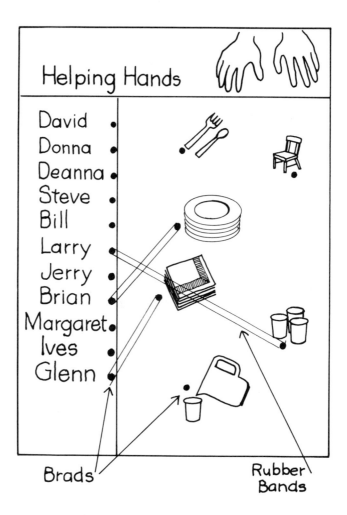

Helping Hands

David
Donna
Deanna
Steve
Bill
Larry
Jerry
Brian
Margaret
Ives
Glenn

Brads

Rubber Bands

on them can indicate the proper placement for flatware, cups, and plates, and each table can be furnished with child-sized pitchers of beverage. Colorful table arrangements with child-made centerpieces serve to heighten the aesthetic appeal of the meal.

As the children seat themselves and pour their beverage, the adult can serve individual plates, unless preserved trays are provided. In some cases, children can be allowed to serve their own plates from "community bowls." Positive social habits are encouraged with this practice, and children are introduced to measurement since they must attend to serving sizes.

Plates should be at least standard in size. Large plates tend to make servings appear to be smaller and less overwhelming to some children who may have poor appetites. Cautious children can be served a "no-thank-you/please" helping of foods that they are unsure of. This serving is, of course, just a tasting portion. When asked if they would like more, they have the option of saying, "No, thank you" or "Yes, please." Their wishes should be respected.

It is important not to overfeed children. Generally, they should be served about one tablespoon for each year of their life from each food group, unless they request more, or less. For example, serving a four-year-old two tablespoons of fruit and two tablespoons of peas would satisfy the requirements for the vegetable and fruit group. Requests for refills should be granted, provided more food is available and provided they have eaten most of the other foods from their plates.

Damp sponges should be available at each table for cleanup in the event of a spill. This practice helps to promote feelings of competence and responsibility for one's own behavior. A whisk broom and dust pan can also be on hand to enable children from each table to team up and share the responsibility of whisking the crumbs away.

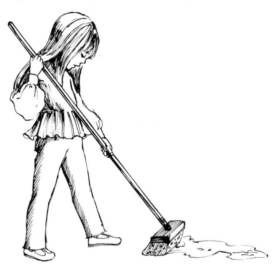

When a child-centered physical environment and a positive emotional climate have been established, the task of feeding young children can become one that brings joy to all who participate. Introducing new foods to children in such an atmosphere is sure to prove a successful venture.

Overcoming Food Prejudices and Introducing New Foods

Children who have a wide range of food likes are more likely to be well nourished than children whose tastes are limited to a few favorites. The child care or preschool setting offers excellent opportunities for expanding the palates of young children.

Supervising adults must have a genuine interest in the nutrition habits of children and also realize that their personal attitudes toward food will influence the eating habits of the children in their care. It is, therefore, helpful to model an adventuresome attitude toward the prospect of exploring new foods and discovering and relishing new tastes and smells.

Below are some tips for motivating even the most cautious young-sters to reach new heights in gustatory experience.

1. Let children help to prepare some of their own foods, particularly if resistance to the food is expected. This technique is discussed fully in Chapter 5.

2. If the food in question is a vegetable or fruit, freeze it into popsicle form. Freezing food slightly modifies the taste. Children will nibble and suck frozen, raw green beans, for example, even though they may have previously found them objectionable in another form.

3. Apply the association principle! Associate a previously disliked or untried food with an interesting dip or spread. This method is especially effective when the dip or spread is made by the children. Try the individual portion recipes for dips in Chapter 5. Children will dip the troublesome vegetable and lick or suck it repeatedly becoming accustomed to it by degree.

4. Give some foods creative names. "Cowboy beans," for example, may be more appealing than pork and beans.

5. Call attention to a fun and appealing property of the food. For example, "Who knows what crunch means?"

6. Cook green vegetables only until they turn bright green. They should still be crunchy. The color and texture are more appealing to children and more vitamins are retained when they are cooked in this way.

7. Cook Brussels sprouts, cauliflower, and cabbage only slightly. Over-cooking increases the sulfurous odors of these vegetables, making them offensive to some children.

8. Use the "no-thank-you/please" tasting portion for cautious children. This leaves the door open for future changes in taste preferences.

9. Serve foods on standard-sized plates. Foods that are suspicious looking to some children will appear less threatening if they are dwarfed by the size of the plate.

10. Explore new foods in informal ways. Some ideas are presented in Chapter 6. One example is to have children grow their own sprouts and eat them in a sandwich or a salad.

11. Give an "I-tasted-a-new-food" badge to those brave children who try an unfamiliar food.

SOME COMMON PITFALLS
TO AVOID

It is always frustrating when children refuse to eat food their bodies need. We know that food is expensive and requires a great deal of effort and care to prepare well. When it is wasted, adults quite naturally feel disappointed and concerned. Self-control is required to maintain a relaxed atmosphere at the table when one feels somewhat responsible for the nutritional intake of children.

It may help to realize, however, that even though it is desirable for children to enjoy a wide variety of foods, some foods, no matter how well planned or presented, will remain only just tolerable to some children, and others will reject them outright.

Adults who become worrisome and prod and nag children to eat will compound existing problems and frequently create new ones.

Below are some pitfalls to avoid when working to improve the diets of young children.

1. Cajoling or giving extra attention for **not** eating only serves to reinforce the unwanted behavior.

2. Threatening with loss of privileges or punishment tempts children to be sneaky. Children have been observed packing their cheeks like chipmunks, only to spit out the hidden food when they thought that no one was looking. Moreover, children frequently engage in a battle of wills at the table because they need to feel in control.

3. Using bribery, especially with desserts or other foods, can condition children to think of food as a reward for good behavior or as a source of comfort. This may lead to overeating in times of emotional stress.

4. Stressing the need for a "clean plate" promotes overeating and distracts the child from paying attention to inner cues which signal satiation.

5. Rushing causes children to become disorganized and promotes stress and overeating. Children should be given plenty of time to chew food well and to have conversation in a relaxed atmosphere. Since people have different rates for eating and digestion, it is reasonable to assume that some children will finish early, while others will appear to dawdle. It may be helpful, therefore, to provide a quiet place with books or puzzles for those children who finish early.

6. Serving meals in the same way, day in and day out, can become monotonous to the children. Look for ways to add variety when this occurs. Some ideas for breaking dull mealtime routines are given in the next section.

**VARIATIONS
ON A MEALTIME THEME**

Young children seem to thrive on routine. They like to know what comes next; knowing makes them feel smart and is reassuring to them. However, sometimes routines can become tiresome and boring. When this happens, children begin to "act out" their need for novel stimulation by engaging in misbehavior. Falling out of a chair on purpose, for example, becomes more interesting that sitting in it every day at the same time and place. Adults also find an occasional break from the daily routine to be stimulating.

Many exciting variations in the mealtime setting are possible. The possibilities are limited only by the imagination of the adults who are responsible for planning and serving meals. Below are some suggestions for spicing up a dull lunch or snacktime routine.

Fancy Dress Day. Have a dress-up day. Decorate placemats and make paper flower centerpieces. Play soft music and dim the lights. Get ready for this important day by practicing good manners through role play in the housekeeping center.

Grandperson's Day. Children who have no grandparents can share with other children. Prepare a special friendship song or finger play to perform for the special guests.

You plan it. Let the children in each group have a turn planning a menu from the basic four food groups. The cook can supervise the planning session.

Serve family style. Place one or two bowls, partly filled, on the table and allow the children to serve themselves. Gradually increase the number of bowls until the children are able to serve all of their own foods. Specify the appropriate amount for each serving. Let the children practice serving.

Turn about. Let the children, perhaps with the aid of a few parents or senior citizen volunteers, prepare a snack for the cooks. Set the "special persons'" table with a fancy cloth and centerpiece or make a corsage for them.

Buffet style. Serve the meal buffet style. Practice scooping serving sizes in the sand table or in a container of dried rice or beans beforehand.

Play restaurant. Make a menu chart by using picture symbols for each food, and make "order forms" with the same symbols on them. One child from each group of four children can play the role of the waiter or waitress and take orders while the "cooks" dish up the portions.

Have a picnic. Spread an old parachute on the grass. Eat a snack or a bag lunch on it. Afterwards, play a parachute game together, scattering the crumbs for the birds and little animals that live in the grass.

Have a cookout. Cook over a campfire. (Be sure there is adequate adult supervision and a fire extinguisher handy for this one.) This activity is particularly appealing in the spring when children are interested in talking about vacations.

Here's how: Set up a tent or two outside (improvise if necessary.) Beg or borrow backpacks, coolers, and a few sleeping bags. Take along a plastic garbage bag for trash. Plan to cook lunch or at least snack, and

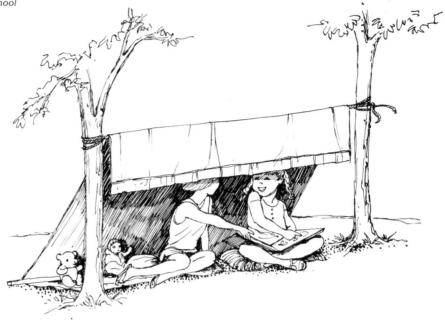

stay out for as long as possible. Be sure to have enough activities planned to keep everyone busy. Fill the backpacks with activities. Some children will want to pretend to sleep in the tents, and others will role play other camping adventures.

The campfood should be nutritious—raw fruit or vegetables, trail mixes of dried fruit and nuts, and whole-wheat sandwiches are a few suggestions. Avoid taking candy, potato chips, soda pops, or sugared drink mixes.

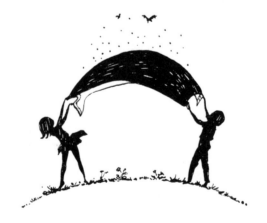

Plate decoration party. Children may decorate their own plates by using professional decorating instruments like the "super shooter." Fill the instrument with mashed potatoes and, presto! A fancy border can be made to encircle the plate. Rosettes can be made with cooked sweet potatoes, pureed liver, peanut butter, or cooked pumpkin.

Prepare an around-the-world menu. Schedule an ethnic food for snack or mealtime every few weeks. To "get in the mood" for the treat, plan ways to add atmosphere to the setting. For example, before serving sukiyaki, a Japanese dish, explore other aspects of the Japanese culture like origami, block printing, or kimono making.

Kimonos can be improvised by cutting arm and neck holes in pillowcases and opening the front from top to bottom. Children can tie-dye them by bunching the fabric, fastening the "wads" with plastic clips or rubberbands, and dipping them into a cold-water-dye. When dried, the kimonos can be worn to the meal.

Decorate the lunch area with Oriental art, child-made drawings, and perhaps prints borrowed from the library, and play recorded Oriental music to create an "authentic" atmosphere. Reinforcement activities of this kind can help to turn a simple meal or snack into an "occasion."

Bag lunches. Bag lunches can be made nutritious if the typical "bag fare" of chips and sweets is avoided. They can be taken on a walking field trip, eaten on the playground, or just taken outside.

Field trips. Go shopping and buy food for a snack or lunch. Some field trip possibilities include fish markets, farmers' markets, grocery stores, fruit and vegetable stands, and pumpkin or peanut patches.

REVIEW ACTIVITIES

1. Visit a preschool or child care center during lunch.
   a. Describe the physical setting.
   b. Describe the emotional climate.
   c. How did the children respond to each item on the menu?
   d. What suggestions given in this chapter could be used to interest the children in trying some of the least preferred items?
   e. Did you observe adults using cajolery, bribery, or threats to get children to eat? Describe.
2. If you work at a center or nursery school, choose one of the suggestions given in this chapter for varying the lunchtime setting and implement it. Take pictures of the event and mount them in a scrapbook. Record and include the children's dictated and illustrated accounts of the event. Read their book to them and share it with the parents.

chapter four

preparing **FOOD**
with young children

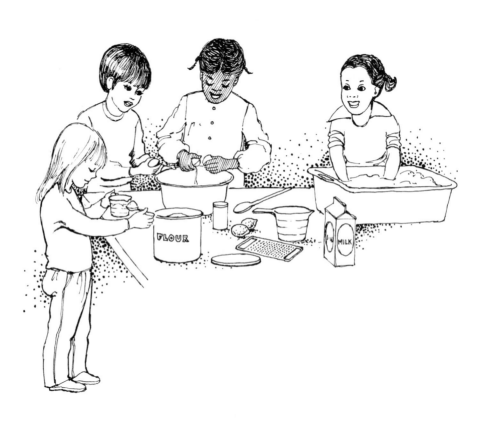

OBJECTIVES

After reading this chapter the reader will be able to:

- Prepare picture recipes for children who have not yet learned to read.
- Use cooking as a means of introducing children to unfamiliar foods and nutrition concepts.
- Create a snack center where young children can prepare their own snacks independently.

"I don't eat worms," wailed Willie when he was served chow mein for lunch at the center. "My mommie won't let me," he protested further.

"They aren't worms. They're noodles and sprouts, Willie," his teacher replied. "They're good for you. They'll make you grow."

"I don't like them."

"Have you ever tried chow mein before?"

"No."

"How do you know you won't like it then?"

"They're all mixed up," he whined.

"Just try a little taste," she urged.

"I don't want to."

"You can have your pudding when you've tasted it."

(Silence)

Getting children to try food that appears unappetizing to them or that they already decided to dislike can turn dining areas into battlefields. When bribery and cajolery are used to try to force children to overcome their food prejudices, most youngsters set their heels firmly, and their dislikes become entrenched. Power struggles ensue and neither party wins with this approach.

New foods, even previously disliked foods, can be presented to preschoolers in ways that make them practically irresistible. One of the most effective means of luring cautious youngsters into risking a taste trauma is to allow them to help prepare the food in question. When resistance to a certain food is anticipated, presenting it in this way increases the chances that the food will at least be tasted by the child. Interest is piqued and motivation to try the food is heightened at each stage of its preparation.

Preparing food with children is an activity that capitalizes on the informal structure of the early childhood setting and the investigative nature of young children. It encourages children with previously limited food experiences to "discover" new tastes, smells, and nutrients that they may be missing at home, thus improving the quality of their food intake. This method also provides a means of incorporating nutrition education into the early childhood curriculum. This letter to parents describing a cooking experience provides an illustration.

Dear Parents,
When we cooked pizza together, we

NUTRITION	Learned that pizza is made by combining many different foods that are good for our bodies. These foods are good for you whether eaten separately or mixed together.
SCIENCE	*Predicted, observed,* and *described* what happened to the ingredients when we combined and cooked them.
MATH	*Counted* pepperoni slices, and cut them in *quarters* before we put them on the pizza. We used real money to purchase the ingredients at the store. As we worked, we used math terms such as *more, less, enough, too much, as much as,* and *equal.*
LANGUAGE ARTS	a. Used *classification skills* to find the necessary items at the grocery store.
	b. *Followed directions.* The directions were illustrated on a recipe symbol chart.
	c. Used *visual discrimination* skills to match the labels on the items we bought at the store.
	d. *Dictated and illustrated* an experience story. Our language was stimulated during the cooking activity. We heard and used new terms in meaningful context. We were introduced to the idea of "ethnic foods."
MOTOR SKILLS	*Stirred, poured,* and *sifted.* This gave us fine and gross motor practice needed for learning to write.
ART	Discussed shapes, textures, and colors.
SOCIAL STUDIES	a. Were introduced to the *economic system* when we visited the grocery store to purchase the ingredients.
	b. *Shared* the experience with our classmates.
	c. Learned to *work together.* Each member had a responsibility for a different part of the project. We helped to organize the project.
	d. Developed *respect* for the food preferences and ideas of others.

Frequently child's play appears frivolous to those who are unaware of the child's need to have first-hand experience to learn. Obviously, the children who participated in this experience were not only being introduced to pepperoni and various kinds of cheeses but were developing many other skills and concepts as well. Cooking pizza merely provided the vehicle for this learning to take place.

The task of learning to use tools for measuring time and ingredients (clocks, timers, spoons, and cups) was made more meaningful because the goal was a "real" one, resulting in an edible product. Pencil and paper approaches in these and other concept areas are poor substitutes for the kind of active involvement that can be experienced while cooking with children.

SNACK AND COOKING CENTERS

The preparation of food by children is considered by some adults to be so important that creative food experiences are a regularly scheduled activity. In many classrooms, special areas called *snack centers* and *cooking centers* are created by teachers to provide for this activity. Few learning centers offer more varied and stimulating opportunities for real, lasting learning than these. The activities presented in these centers can be used to reinforce concepts in all areas of the curriculum. And they can be used with equal success at home, in most child care programs, and in schools.

Although snack and cooking centers have much in common, there are some fundamental differences in the ways they are set up and managed and in the kind and quality of the experiences that can be had by the children who visit them.

The Cooking Center

Children who visit the cooking center, usually under the direction of an adult, may prepare a snack there or perhaps a dish to be included in the noon meal. Sometimes the cooking center is used to prepare a treat for a special occasion or to provide a means of introducing or reinforcing concepts from curriculum areas (for example, the mathematical concept of measurement or the language arts skill of symbol reading with the aid of picture recipe charts). Adults who regularly incorporate the cooking center in the curriculum are able to capitalize on the naturally active learning styles of children and are therefore ensured a higher level of involvement by the children.

Family home caregivers and parents have ready-made cooking centers. With only a few modifications, they can begin to use the versatile medium of cooking. Setting up a cooking center from "scratch" in a school classroom or a child care center, however, requires a little more planning and ingenuity.

CREATING A COOKING CENTER

A hotplate is an ample substitute for a stove top. It may even be an improvement over the stove, because it can be placed at a level that is low enough for children to observe the action of heat on the ingredients. Since a hotplate, an electric crockpot, or skillet will probably be used for most cooking projects, the center should be located near an outlet, preferably in a low-traffic area of the room. The hotplate should be on a low table near a wall so that children will not trip over the cord. Safety is a primary consideration in all activities where heat, electricity, and sharp implements are to be used with children.

To protect the children from the burners and to anchor the hotplate firmly, place it inside a shallow crate with sides that are only slightly higher than the level of the burner. One side of the crate, the side from which the adult will work, can be removed to provide access to the knobs and pot handles. (Pot handles should always be turned *AWAY* from children.) The other side of the crate should be low enough to allow easy viewing by the children.

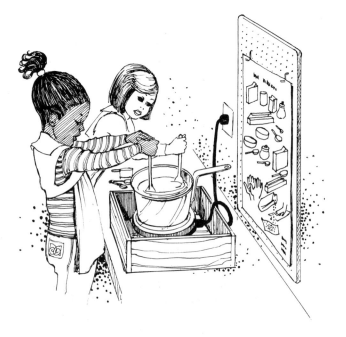

A shelf should be placed near the table for the purpose of providing storage for cooking utensils and ingredients. The shelf should be low enough to allow children access to the materials so they can participate in organizing the activity.

Stocking the shelves with the necessary equipment requires planning in the initial stages. A list of supplies should be made and a source for them found. Parents may want to help with this project. Because most parents work and have little time to volunteer, they often welcome opportunities to become involved in other ways. Frequently, a letter of request explaining the function of the cooking center and describing how cooking can be used to reinforce social and academic skills will result in donations of many of the supplies that are needed. Occasionally a blender, beater, or a special spice will have to be brought from home to complete a special project, but if the basic supplies are collected and organized in advance, planning a cooking activity will seem less overwhelming. When most of the supplies and utensils are in place, the adult can move to the next step—planning.

PLANNING THE COOKING EXPERIENCE

The first step in planning a cooking experience is to identify a goal. Ask the question, what do I hope the children will learn from this experience? It is true that many skills and concepts will spontaneously develop during the course of the activity, but it is important for the adult to identify at least one major goal to serve as a focal point for the activity. Goal identification is a major step in planning, because without goals, activities frequently lack direction. Some appropriate goals to use while cooking with young children are given in Chapter 5.

To select a goal that is interesting to young children and is also appropriate for their developmental levels, one must first observe the children. Activities that evolve from the naturally expressed questions of children rather than from structured, adult-directed questions will more easily motivate young children.

With motivation heightened, a project can easily be initiated that will enable the children to accomplish the goal set by the adult. For example, to enable the children to learn how to *observe* and *describe* the changes that occur when heat is applied to some foods, the children could be provided with opportunities to examine a raw egg, to boil it, and to eat it at snacktime. This activity could be followed by letting the children dictate a letter to the teacher to be sent to the parent who donated the eggs, describing what happened to the eggs when they were boiled. All of the new terms and words learned by the children during the experience could be included in the letter.

The project could be further enhanced by providing other experiences with eggs, perhaps making egg salad while using a picture recipe for the children to follow during the activity. Picture recipe charts should be used whenever possible in the preparation of food. They are important teaching tools for some of the reasons outlined here. Picture recipe charts

1. Enable children to begin to see how spoken words and ideas can be represented graphically with pictures and word symbols
2. Encourage children to follow directions
3. Promote symbol reading from "top to bottom, left to right"
4. Provide a record of the experience that can be reviewed
5. Illustrate the need for following a sequence to accomplish a goal
6. Encourage children to become independent and develop initiative

77   Preparing a picture recipe chart is not difficult. The picture symbols used

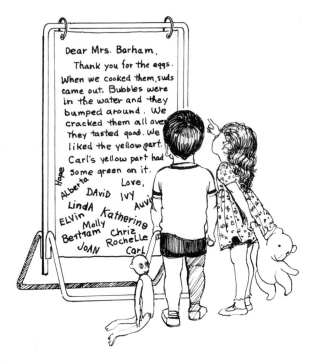

The letter on the chart reads:

Dear Mrs. Barham,

Thank you for the eggs. When we cooked them, suds came out. Bubbles were in the water and they bumped around. We cracked them all over. They tasted good. We liked the yellow part. Carl's yellow part had some green on it.

Love,
Hope, Alberta, David, Ivy, Linda, Auvi, Elvin, Katherine, Molly, Bertram, Chriz, Rochelle, Joan, Carl

in them, like the written symbols in our culture, should be arbitrarily agreed upon by the group. The adult merely says, "This circle stands for an orange," for example. One doesn't have to be an artist to make an orange symbol that children can "read," or symbols for a cup or spoon that are discernible. Younger children may need more "lifelike" representations of ingredients, like magazine pictures or actual box labels. Older children, however, will benefit from interpreting the more abstract symbols that are spontaneously drawn by the adult. Some suggestions for preparing a picture recipe chart are as follows:

1. Use as many real objects (labels, boxes, containers) as possible on the chart. They can be glued or fastened with brads or hooks. This helps children begin to "bridge the gap" between objects, picture symbols, and written words.

2. Minimize the amount of print that appears on the chart. When word symbols are used, they should be printed neatly, clearly, and in correct manuscript form.

3. Avoid visual clutter. Include only a few steps on each chart, spacing between groups of objects and symbols.

4. When possible, use the same sequence for all recipes. This allows children to see consistencies in printed words and other symbol forms. (See Chapter 5 for examples of picture recipe charts.)

GETTING THE ACTIVITY UNDERWAY

Cooking activities are rarely suitable for large group participation. In centers and classrooms the project should be introduced to the whole group during circle time or during the morning opening activity period when the group is together, but it should be carried out later in smaller groups. During circle time, a story, song, or finger play related to the project can be used to motivate the group for the activity. This is also a good time to read the recipe chart together, explain the system that will be used to schedule the children into the cooking area, discuss safety rules, and assign responsibility for cleanup.

Some children can be rotated into the cooking center while others work elsewhere in the room. If it is determined, however, that the whole group is to participate in the cooking activity at the same time, the children should be divided into teams of four or five so that each child will have an opportunity to participate, not merely watch. For some projects, like soup making, it may be necessary to provide each team with an adult supervisor. That person should be given a recipe and briefed on the objectives that are to be accomplished during the project. For example: Each child will learn to scrub, peel, and dice a potato.

All the ingredients and utensils that will be used in the activity should be assembled on trays and ready to use. The recipe should be prominently displayed so the children can see it and begin to work without delay.

At the beginning of the activity, safety rules should be discussed. If sharp tools are to be used, procedures for using them carefully should be demonstrated by the adult. Then, the children should, in turn, demonstrate their ability to use the instruments safely before they are allowed to proceed with the activity.

There are a few other small, but important, details to attend to before beginning a cooking activity with young children. To ensure a successful experience, review this list.

1. Do you have a plan for introducing the activity to the group?
2. Are the ingredients and necessary utensils in place?
3. Are picture recipes posted?
4. Did you break the recipe down into small units to maximize participation by the children?
5. Do the children know what to do when it is not their turn to cook?
6. Have safety precautions been taken?
7. Will you have enough time to complete the project in a relaxed manner?
8. How many children will work at the station at one time?
9. Do the children know what they are to do when they finish at the cooking center?
10. Have you planned follow-up activities?
11. Are sponges available for cleanup?
12. Have you considered all of the possibilities for learning?
13. Are you relaxed enough to enjoy the experience, settle back, and observe the children?

When you have seen to all of these details you are ready to begin the activity. Item 13 in the checklist is particularly important because the cooking experience should not be entirely adult-directed. The adult's role is to provide the opportunity, materials, encouragement, and some direction, and then to observe the children's responses and interact appropriately with them. It is important to remember that the quality of the product is of less importance than the process of preparing it together.

Listening to Learn About Children's Thinking

It is necessary for the adult to *listen* to children as they express their thoughts while working together in the cooking center. Adults often become so involved in teaching and talking that they interfere with the thought processes of the child and fail to hear how children are responding to the activity. Instead of "feeding" children with a steady stream of facts, it is more appropriate to stimulate thought by asking divergent questions like: "What do you think will happen if we put this into the oven?" The child who responds that the batter will "turn into a cake" when it is placed in the oven reveals a level of thinking that is characteristic of the preoperational child as defined by Piaget (1964). Adults who listen carefully to children as they work gain insights that enable them to adjust the level of instruction to meet the developmental needs of children. A perceptive adult might notice, for example, that some of the children who helped to bake bread failed to connect the loaf that magically appeared in the oven and the batter they initially placed there. The lack of reversibility and limited ability to comprehend transformations prior to age of six or seven make it difficult for young children to understand that, although a change has taken place in the appearance of the batter, the basic ingredients remain, and that the bread or cake in question did not "magically" replace the batter while it was out of sight in the oven.

The adult, upon discovering children who are functioning at this developmental level, should plan additional opportunities that will allow them to observe the action of heat upon ingredients. Glass pots and low tables for cooking are but two adjustments that could be made to maximize opportunities for observing change in motion. And by retracing the process, using the symbol recipe, the child's understanding of the event can be further enhanced.

Understanding that food undergoes change when subjected to varying temperatures or when mixed with either wet or dry ingredients lays the foundation for understanding the chemical changes that food undergoes when it is absorbed and used by our bodies. Children need repeated experiences of this nature more than they need to be drilled on nutrition facts.

Other remarks made by the children such as, "We gotta take the crust off the orange first" or "The egg has oil in it," contain clues that aid the adult in selecting appropriate follow-up activities. The child who thinks that egg whites are oil, for example, should be provided with opportunities to examine oil closely and to compare the oil with the white of an egg by taste, texture, and as many ways as possible. Moreover, experiences with other ingredients that look alike but have different properties will further encourage observation and classification skills in young children (salt, sugar, talcum powder, flour).

Like cooking centers, snack centers provide children with opportunities for developing skills and concepts that are prerequisites for later, more advanced nutrition concepts. And like cooking centers, snack centers can be used to improve the nutritional intake of young children.

The Snack Center

The snack center is designed to allow children to "assemble" their own food at snacktime without cooking it. Ideally, it should be made available to children near midmorning or midafternoon and used like any other activity center. As the children (two or three at a time) finish their projects, they should put away their materials, wash their hands, and go to the snack center where they prepare and eat their snacks. At the center, they may sit with a few friends, share conversation, and otherwise enjoy their food, after which they clean up the crumbs, napkins, and cups to make way for other children. In the snack center, adult supervision should be minimized to encourage responsibility and independence in young children.

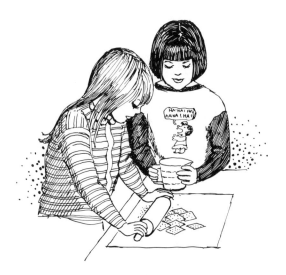

Adults who use snack centers that serve only a few children at a time report that this system helps to improve the nutritional intake of the children because they are directly involved in the preparation of their own food. Moreover, this approach also eliminates many of the discipline problems that otherwise occur when the traditional method of serving snacks to a whole group at one time is employed. This is because, when snack centers are used, children do not have to wait for uncomfortable periods of time to be served, a situation that frequently *creates* discipline problems. Moreover, the activities of other children are not interrupted, resulting in less wasted time by adults and children and fewer opportunities for negative exchanges between adult and child. As a bonus, children begin to view themselves as competent individuals. After all, preparing one's own food independently is a real grown-up task!

Parents can make a snack center by making food available to children on the bottom shelf of the refrigerator or a cabinet that is easily accessible.

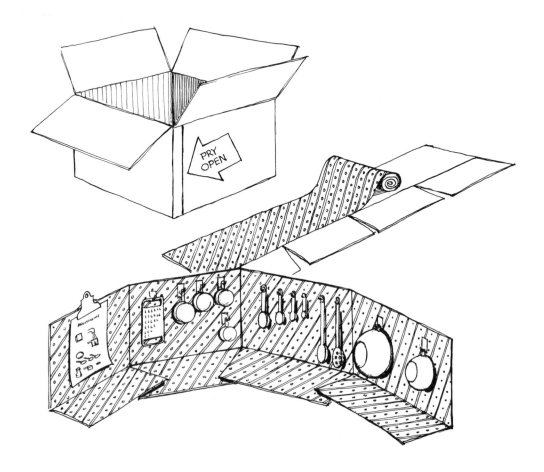

There are some important management problems that must receive special attention before this method can be successfully implemented. Some suggestions follow.

1. Try this approach with children who are four years of age or older. It can be used on a limited basis with some three-year-old groups, but younger groups will require more supervision.

2. Prior to opening the snack center each day, the adult should instruct the children concerning the procedure to be followed. This can be done during opening exercises, so that only a brief reminder is necessary when the center is actually opened. Sample directions might include, "There are enough crackers for each person to have two," or "Remember, only the spreader goes into the peanut butter jar, never fingers!" or "Please wipe the peanut butter off the spreader with your toast, not with your fingers." Remember to minimize talking in order to maintain their interest and ensure that main points are understood.

3. Plan snacks that can be prepared with little or no adult supervision after they are introduced (some examples are given in Chapter 5).

4. Whenever possible, post a symbol recipe in the center for the children to follow.

5. Plan only nutritious snacks. Children need to make *all* of their food intake count. Since their stomachs are small, space should not be taken with food that is low in nutritional value.

6. Post a "Wash Your Hands, Please" sign at the center.

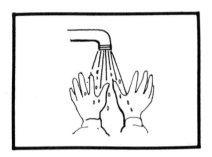

7. The snack center should be opened at about the same time every day for about 30 to 40 minutes. This amount of time will allow children to "work it into their schedule." It should be closed early enough not to interfere with their appetites for the next meal.

8. The snack table should be freshly scrubbed and laid with a fresh cloth or butcher paper to cover the table.

9. All utensils, vessels, ingredients, napkins, and cups that are needed to prepare and to serve the snack should be on the table or be easily accessible to the children. They should not have to ask for frequent adult assistance.

10. It is important to limit the number of children who can work at the center at one time. This can be done by limiting the number of chairs at the table, providing children with "snack tickets" to mail at the station when they go or by having a limited number of clothespins available for the children to "wear" to the station. Only children with pins on, for example, would be admitted to the station. When children finish, they simply replace the clothespin, perhaps by fastening it to the sign so that it will be available to the next child. With the clothespin system, the adult can vary the number of children who can use the station at one time.

11. Review the management techniques that are discussed in the cooking center section of this chapter.

The preparation of food by children, whether by cooking or by assembling ingredients in a snack center, provides a springboard for learning. Ideas and concepts stimulated in this way can be reinforced and further explored in other curriculum areas. Moreover, by using food as a medium for learning, the adult ensures a meaningful and highly motivating experience for children.

REVIEW ACTIVITIES

1. Choose a recipe from Chapter 5 that has not yet been illustrated.
   a. Make a symbol recipe for it, using the suggestions given in this chapter.
   b. List the possibilities for learning.
   c. Write a plan for presenting the cooking activity to the children. Try out the plan in a child care center or at home with children. The plan should include a system for controlling the number of children who will participate at one time, a motivating activity, a goal, and a follow-up activity. (Appropriate goals are given prior to the recipes in Chapter 5, and ideas for follow-up activities can be found in Chapter 6.) Before getting underway, be sure to review the checklists given in this chapter to ensure a successful experience.
2. Set up a snack center and a system for using it. Take pictures of the children preparing their snacks independently.
3. Write a letter to parents requesting ingredients to be used in a cooking experience. Be sure to explain some of the "academic" benefits of cooking with children. (Use the open letter to parents given in this chapter and the list of curriculum objectives that are outlined in the next chapter for reference.)
4. Keep a record of the snacks that are served in a center or classroom for two weeks. Could any of these snacks be served in a snack center like the one that was described in this chapter?
5. Choose one snack that you observed being served to children in a group setting. Describe how you would have presented it differently, using the techniques that were discussed in this chapter.

SUGGESTED READINGS

BRUNO, J., and P. DANKAN, *Cooking in the Classroom*. Belmont, Calif.: Fearon Publishers, Inc., 1974.

Preparing Food with Young Children

COHL, V., *Science Experiences You Can Eat*. Philadelphia: J.B. Lippin-cott Company, 1973.

Cooking and Eating with Children: A Way to Learn. Washington, D.C.: Association for Childhood Education International, 1981.

CROFT, D.J., and R.D. HESS, *An Activities Handbook for Teachers of Young Children*. Boston: Houghton Mifflin Co., 1980.

GOODWIN, M.T., and G. POLLEN, *Creative Food Experiences for Children*. Washington, D.C.: Center for Science in the Public Interest, 1974.

Parents' Nursery School, *Kids Are Natural Cooks*, Cambridge, Mass, 1974.

chapter five

RECIPES

for learning

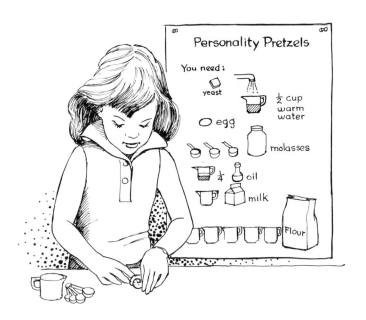

OBJECTIVES

After reading this chapter the reader will be able to:

- Plan and implement a successful cooking activity.
- Organize a cooking activity to promote maximum involvement by the children.
- Justify cooking as a means of integrating all areas of the early childhood curriculum.

If the ultimate nutrition goal is to help children learn to make wise food choices, experiences with food must be planned with that goal in mind. With young children, what we *do* is what we *teach*. Therefore, even the recipes chosen for cooking experiences with children should be chosen with care. Well-chosen recipes are ideal vehicles for learning. They can be used to help children develop behaviors and concepts that are prerequisites for later, more abstract concepts about nutrients and how our bodies use them.

Begin planning for your cooking activity by choosing one of the nutrition goals listed here. Some goals from other areas of the early childhood curriculum follow the nutrition goals. Think of ways to integrate them into your cooking activity also.

NUTRITION EDUCATION GOALS

The child will

- Sample previously untried foods.
- Taste familiar foods prepared in unfamiliar ways.
- Learn the names of unfamiliar foods.
- Describe characteristics of foods discovered through the senses.
- Classify foods (simple classification by color, coverings, and tastes).
- Identify food origins.
- Demonstrate healthy eating habits.
- Plan and select healthful snacks.

- Plan a menu and participate in preparing and serving it.
- Observe food in various stages of change.
- Observe growth of foods.
- Participate in the storage of food (dehydration, canning, and freezing).
- Read recipes to aid in food preparation.
- Meet and interview people who grow, package, and sell food.
- Demonstrate an awareness that food is needed for growth.
- Combine foods to make another food (pizza, stew, soup).
- Discriminate between highly processed, prepackaged foods and foods in their natural states.
- Discuss food commercials seen on television.
- Identify foods with high sugar and salt levels.

INTEGRATING OTHER CURRICULUM GOALS WITH NUTRITION ACTIVITIES

Math. The child will measure ingredients according to the directions given in the recipe. (This requires dividing, assessing quantities, measuring discrete and continous quantities.)

Language Arts. The child will "read" the pictures on the symbol recipe charts to perform the activity in the correct sequence.

Science. The child will observe changes in the properties of the ingredients as they are subjected to extremes in temperature and mixing, will predict outcomes, record "experiments" with foods, describe their properties, and discover cause-and-effect relationships.

Social Studies. The child will cooperate with others to prepare foods and develop executive skills required for organizing and performing a shared project.

Motor Skills. The child will practice fine motor skills required for mixing, pouring, and stirring ingredients.

Art. The child will explore foods through the mediums of painting, printing, drawing, and gluing with a variety of food products.

Music. The child will manipulate foods to determine the sounds that can be made by them and use descriptive terminology like loud, high, low, crunchy, scratchy, rattly, hard, and snapping.

Now look through the recipes in this chapter and the other activities with foods given in Chapter 6 for strategies that can be used to accomplish your chosen goals. To simplify the planning process, use a lesson plan format like the one illustrated in Table 5-1.

Since preparing food with children is an inclusive, integrating activity, many objectives representing all areas of the curriculum can be accomplished simultaneously as evidenced by the lesson plan in Table 5-1. Be

TABLE 5-1 Sample Lesson Plan Format

NUTRITIONAL GOAL	FOOD PREPARATION ACTIVITY	FOOD RELATED ACTIVITY
The child will observe how foods undergo change when ingredients are combined.	Prepare "Miss Muffet's favorite snack."	Make Butter. Visit a dairy.

Other Curriculum Goals:

Language:	To introduce new vocabulary words—curds and whey, liquid, and solid.
Math:	To measure milk and vinegar.
Science:	To separate liquid (whey) from solid (curds) ingredients.

Parent Follow-Up:
Send recipe for cottage cheese home with child.

sure to consider ways to capitalize on the possibilities for learning before presenting cooking activities to children. This is not to say the children should never cook just for the fun of it; enjoyment alone is a desirable goal.

The recipes in this chapter are presented in five sections: (1) Individual Portion, No-Cook Snacks; (2) Dips and Sandwich Spreads; (3) Recipes for the Cooking Center, (4) Foods for Celebrations, and (5) Foods from Many Cultures.

INDIVIDUAL PORTION, NO-COOK SNACKS

The recipes given in this section were developed to allow children to prepare snacks with a minimum of adult intervention. They do not require cooking, and since they are illustrated in individual portions, they can often be mixed by the child in a single bowl or paper cup. The children should be encouraged to try to "figure out" the picture directions on their own. After the first few attempts they will rarely need help.

At the beginning of each recipe the ingredients and utensils needed for the project are shown. This format encourages children to develop organizational skills, since they must check to determine whether they have everything that will be needed to complete the activity before starting. To provide continuity, all recipes should follow the same format.

The adult must purchase the ingredients and make them available, of course. To calculate the amount of each ingredient needed to feed a group of children, first look at the recipe and count the total number of tablespoons required for each ingredient. Now, multiply that number by the number of children to be served, and then read the container label to determine the number of ounces contained in the box or jar of ingredients. Remember that 2 tablespoons equals 1 ounce. Therefore, if the box has 8 ounces of pudding, you can get 16 tablespoons from it. Computation of quantity for large groups is quite simple if you remember these steps.

Giant's Castle

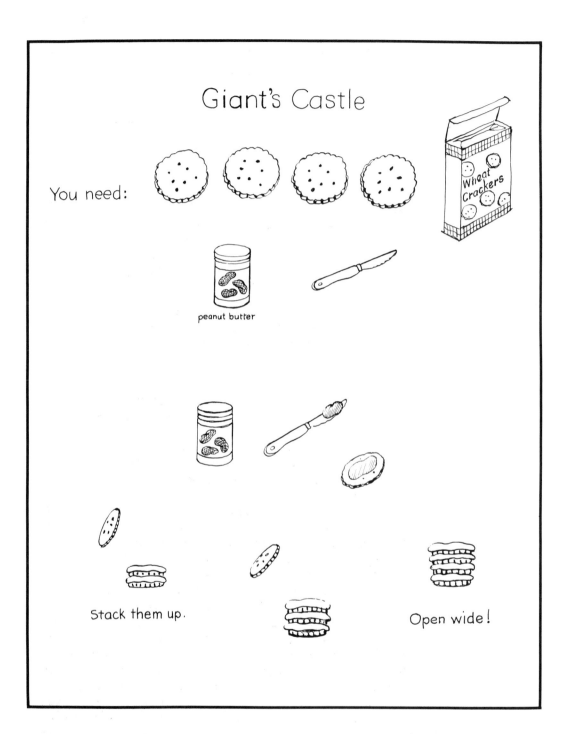

You need:

peanut butter

Stack them up.

Open wide!

Crunchy Munchy

You need:

peanut butter

Raisins

tsp.

¼ tsp.

sesame
seeds

Sunflower
Seeds

¼

Raisins

tsp.

Sunflower
Seeds

tsp.

yum-yum

Fruit Pop

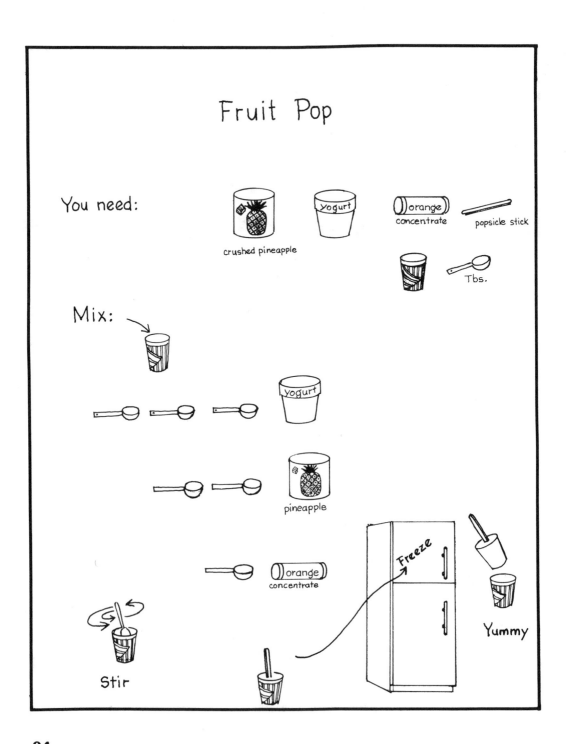

You need:

crushed pineapple

yogurt

orange concentrate

popsicle stick

Tbs.

Mix:

yogurt

pineapple

orange concentrate

Freeze

Stir

Yummy

Yum Kabob

Cut

Spear

chunky pineapple

orange

Raisins

Cider Sipper

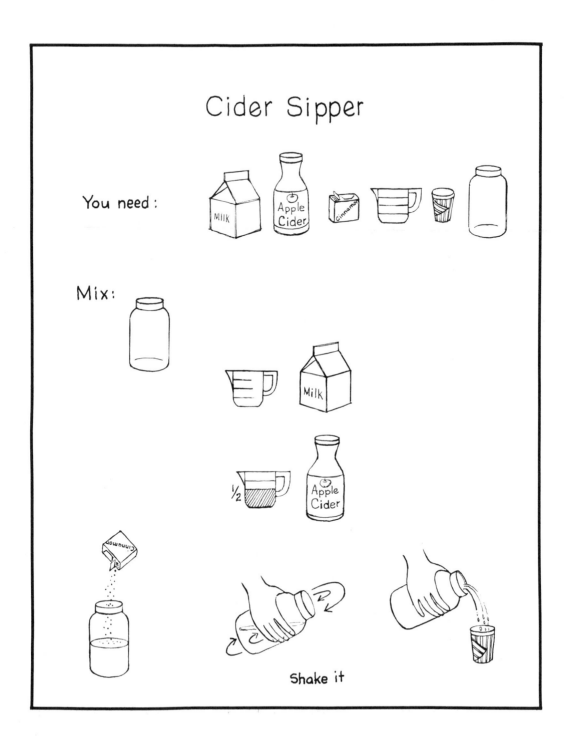

You need:

Mix:

Shake it

Shake and Make

You need:

Peel

Cut

Shake

Butter

whipping cream

cream

You need:

Shake

. . . and shake some more

Droid Salad

You need: cherry 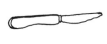 ½

pineapple ring

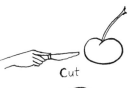 Cut

½

 Peel

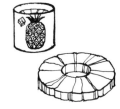

Bugs on a Stick

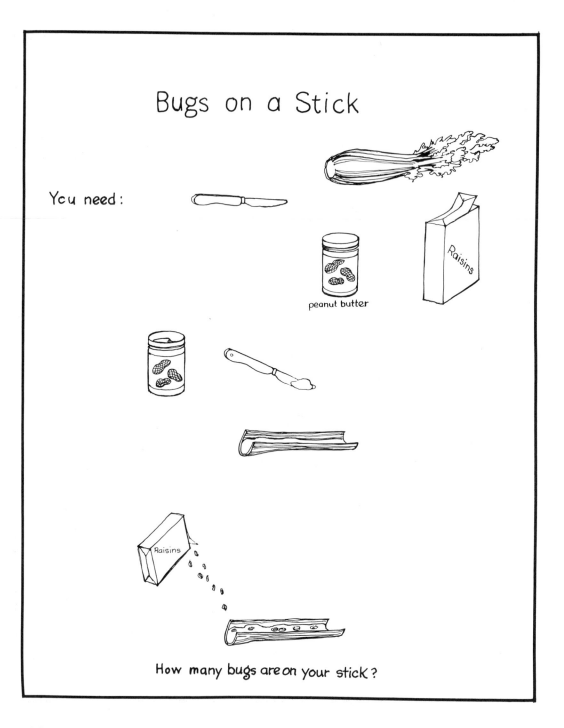

You need:

peanut butter

Raisins

Raisins

How many bugs are on your stick?

Lincoln Logs

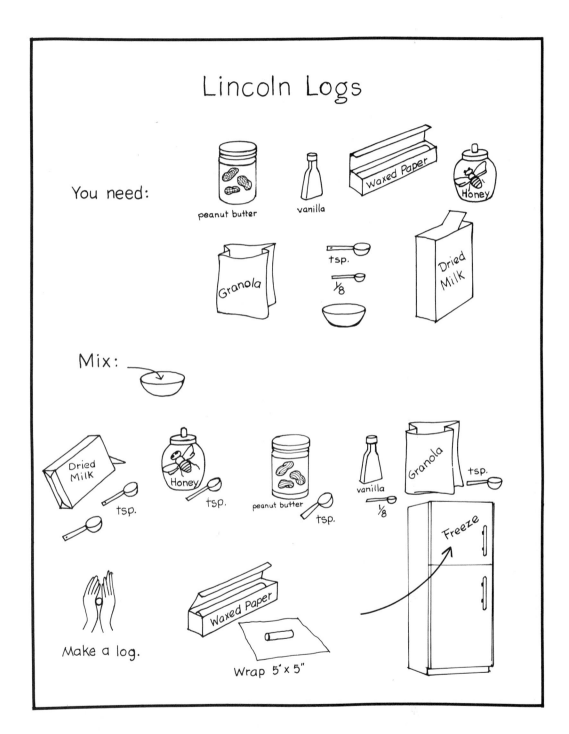

You need:

peanut butter

vanilla

Waxed Paper

Honey

Granola

tsp.

⅛

Dried Milk

Mix:

Dried Milk

tsp.

tsp.

Honey

tsp.

peanut butter

tsp.

vanilla

⅛

Granola

tsp.

Freeze

Make a log.

Waxed Paper

Wrap 5" x 5"

101

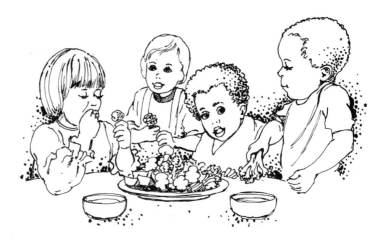

DIPS AND SANDWICH SPREADS

Both spreads and dips are good on vegetables and fruit. Try peanut butter, for example, on bananas, orange slices, zucchini, and even pineapple! Don't impose your prejudices on the children by limiting their offerings to what you think would taste good to you. Children often surprise us with creative combinations. Some foods for dipping, freezing, or spreading are

Fresh Fruits	*Dried Fruits*	*Raw Vegetables*
apple wedges	apricots	carrot sticks
bananas	pitted dates	celery sticks
berries	prunes	cucumber
cantaloupe	pears	cauliflower
kumquats	peaches	cabbage
orange slices	bananas	avocado
grapes	raisins	turnips
mangoes	figs	radishes
pear slices		tomato wedges
peaches		green beans
pineapple sticks		endive
plums		onions
		zucchini
		broccoli
		mushrooms

Other Foods
cheese wedges
waffles
pancakes
crackers
all kinds of bread sticks
toast
biscuits

Many of the foods listed above can be frozen to make "veggie" or fruit pops. Freezing slightly modifies the taste of the food and often makes it more acceptable to children. For teething toddlers, frozen veggie or bread sticks feel good to tender gums.

Combinations suggested in this section can be used as dips or as spreads for crackers or breads. To enable children to prepare their own sandwiches or spread their own crackers, illustrate a simple recipe on an index card or chart paper and display it in the work area. See the recipes "The Giant's Castle" and "Crunchy Munchy" in the previous section for examples of how sandwich making can be illustrated.

Breads for sandwiches should be whole-grain, if possible, rather than white. Whole-grain breads and crackers provide fiber, which has been found to be lacking in the diets of many children. Pumpernickel, pita, and rye are also popular choices with children, in addition to being nutritious.

Often it is difficult to think of ways to break out of the peanut-butter-and-jelly rut. Parents need help with this problem also and would be delighted to receive some of the following ideas for sandwich variety, perhaps in a newsletter! Other ideas for packing sandwiches in bag lunches are included in the first section of Chapter 7.

PEANUT BUTTER

Mix with molasses, chopped nuts, toasted sesame seeds, fruits, shredded carrots, wheat germ, coconut, applesauce, or apple butter.

HOMEMADE MAYONNAISE

Beat 1 egg yolk with 1 teaspoon mustard. Slowly dribble about 1 tablespoon vegetable oil into mixture while beating at medium speed. Then, beat in ½ teaspoon vinegar followed by ½ to 1 cup vegetable oil, also mixed in very slowly. For a thin mayonnaise, add a little more vinegar. To make it stiffer, add more oil.

MEATS

1. Chopped turkey or chicken combined with chopped nuts and celery or pineapple, or mayonnaise and shredded spinach or greens.
2. Beef with mayonnaise or salad dressing and shredded greens.
3. Tuna combined with salad dressing, celery, chopped nuts, apples, and raisins.

EGGS

Chop and mix a hard-boiled egg with mayonnaise or salad dressing and any combination of the following ingredients: celery, raisins, chicken, carrot, sprouts, chopped raw or frozen cooked spinach, cheese, or lettuce.

CHEESE

Mix cottage cheese with any of the following: sesame or caraway seeds, chopped fruit, nuts, applesauce, or tomatoes and cucumbers.

Grate cheddar cheese and mix with salad dressing and chopped nuts or seeds (sesame, pumpkin, or sunflower).

BEANS

Mash and mix with chili sauce and finely chopped onions.

GREEN PEAS

Mash and mix with mayonnaise and finely chopped onions.

VEGETABLE MIX

Thaw frozen peas and mix them, uncooked, with grated carrots, raisins, and mayonnaise.

SPINACH SPREAD OR DIP

Cook a box of frozen spinach, drain, and squeeze out excess water. Mix with 2 cups mayonnaise, half of a finely chopped onion and a little lemon juice.

RECIPES FOR
THE COOKING CENTER

The recipes given in this section should also be illustrated in symbol form, if possible. As guides, use the recipes in the Individual Portion, No-Cook Snacks section of this chapter and follow the directions given in Chapter 4 for illustrating recipes. If the group is large, the tasks should be divided so that teams of children can work on separate parts of the project, combining their work only in the final stages. The recipes in this section are followed by examples of activities which can be used to extend or to reinforce sme of the skills and concepts developed during the cooking activity.

To ensure a successful experience, review the directions for cooking with children given in Chapter 4 before beginning the cooking activity.

PANCAKES

2 cups whole-wheat or buckwheat flour	2 eggs
3 teaspoons baking powder	1½ cups milk
¼ cup toasted wheat germ	3 tablespoons oil
	1 teaspoon molasses

1. Beat eggs well; add milk, molasses, and oil.

2. Let children combine dry ingredients and add them to the mixture. Be careful; don't overmix.

3. Let the children help to dribble the batter through a funnel onto a greased electric frying pan. The batter might take the shape of their initial or a new letter name. When bubbles appear on the surface, the pancake is ready to be turned.

4. Serve with a topping of any of the following: chopped nuts, apple butter, applesauce, fruit, grated carrots, yogurt, sour cream, and raisins. Makes about three dozen very small pancakes.

Extended activities: Make up a story about a pancake man and his adventures. This story might resemble the one about the Ginger

Bread Man. Or write an experience story and have the children illustrate it. Read the story *Pancakes for Breakfast.*[1]

SNACK STICKS

1 cup cornmeal
¼ cup wheat germ
5 tablespoons sesame seeds
1 tablespoon vegetable herb
   seasoning
3 tablespoons safflower oil

4-ounce container of
unsweetened Dannon yogurt,
or other yogurt with active
cultures
3 sheets waxed paper

1. Preheat oven to 375° F.

2. Let the children mix dry ingredients.

3. Blend oils with yogurt, and mix with dry ingredients.

4. Form dough into four small balls, place each on a sheet of waxed paper 12 by 12 inches, cover with second sheet, and roll out dough.

5. Remove the top paper, and let the children practice measurement skills by cutting the dough into 1 by 2 inches in size.

6. Invert the paper onto a cookie sheet, remove paper, and bake for about 15 minutes.
Serves about 12 children.

Extended activities: Try making yogurt or some other foods that come from milk.

CIRCLE BREAD

2 cups sifted whole-wheat pastry flour
3¾ teaspoons baking powder
⅓ cup oil
¼ cup milk

1. Allow the children to sift and mix the dry ingredients.

2. Gradually add the milk and oil. Mix slightly.

3. Divide the dough into two balls, sprinkle the table with flour, and let the children knead and roll out the dough to about ¼ inch thick. Cut dough with anything that will make a circle shape. (Vary with seasonal cutters or animal- or letter-shaped cookie cutters.) Fry in a lightly greased electric pan on low heat. When biscuits rise, turn them over. Makes about 20.

Extended activities: Find circles in the room. Make a chart of round things. Repeat activity with other shapes. A trip to a farm or zoo followed by making "animal bread" would be fun.

PRETZEL INITIALS

1 package dry yeast
½ cup warm water
1 egg
3 tablespoons molasses

¼ cup cooking oil
1 cup milk
5 cups flour

[1]T. de Pavola, *Pancakes for Breakfast* (New York: Harcourt Brace Jovanovich, 1978).

1. Let the children sprinkle the yeast in the water and stir until it dissolves.

2. Separate the egg yolk from the white and mix the yolk with molasses, oil, milk, and yeast. Add enough flour to make the dough stiff and easy to handle.

3. Divide the dough into four small balls, and let the children knead the balls on a floured surface for about five minutes before rolling them out.

4. Let the dough balls rise for about an hour before letting the children cut them into inch wide strips to form the shape of their initials, snakes, snails, or other objects d'art.

5. Place these on a cookie sheet, brush with egg white, and sprinkle with Parmesan or coarse salt.

6. Bake at 425° F for about 20 minutes. They should be golden brown and chewy. Makes about two dozen.

Extended activities: Before beginning the activity, pour a package of dry yeast and ½ cup warm water and 2 tablespoons sugar into a jar. Stir, and fasten a rubber surgical glove over the opening of the jar. During the cooking experience, the children can watch the progress of the glove as the gases inflate it. Ask the children if they think their dough might also become inflated. Follow up by letting the children dramatize the expanding yeast by "puffing up" their bodies.

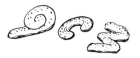

THE MUFFIN MAN'S FAVORITE

1 cups sifted whole-wheat flour	1 cup milk
¼ cup wheat germ	1 egg
1 tablespoon baking powder	¼ cup shortening
¼ cup molasses	

1. Preheat oven to 400° F.

2. Let children sift flour, beat egg, measure and melt shortening, and grease the muffin tins.

3. Talk about which ingredients are wet and which are dry. Combine the dry ingredients.

4. Combine the milk, egg, and molasses, and stir them into the dry ingredients.

5. Add shortening and stir lightly. Leave some lumps.

6. Fill the muffin tins about three-fourths full.

7. Set a timer for about 12 minutes and bake the muffins. If small tins are used, the recipe makes about 2 dozen. In the larger tins, it makes about a dozen, and the muffins will need to bake a little longer.

Extended activities: Learn the song about the muffin man. Talk about what the term *dozen* means.

PIZZA MIAS

 1 *teaspoon garlic salt*
 1 *teaspoon Italian seasoning*
 15-ounce can of tomato sauce
 8 *toasted English muffins, halved*
 cheeses, sausages, salami, onions, olives, green peppers,
 mushrooms, pepperoni, and so forth

1. Preheat oven to 450° F.

2. The children can mix the tomato sauce, garlic salt, and Italian seasoning; chop all the vegetables; and slice the meats. Slices of salami can be quartered and sausages sliced and then halved (a good measurement activity).

3. Let each child spread 1 tablespoon sauce on the muffin of their choice and choose the ingredients they want to sprinkle on their pizzas.

4. Place in oven until done or place under a broiler for a few minutes. If the broiler is used, you may want to preheat the sauce a little.

Extended activities: Allow the children to investigate each of the ingredients separately. Let them guess what the tomato sauce is made from. What other foods are made with tomato sauce? Make some catsup by mixing tomato paste, a little lemon juice, and sugar. Use the catsup for a snacktime dip the next day.

INCREDIBLE EDIBLE

 1 *box old-fashioned oats*
 ⅓ *cup boiling water*
 ⅓ *cup molasses*
 ⅓ *cup vegetable oil*
 ½ *cup peanuts (optional)*

1. Let the children pour the oats into a large bowl.

2. Mix in boiling water, molasses, and oil. Stir until oats are covered, then spread on a cookie sheet.

3. Bake for 15 minutes at 300° F, stir, and bake for about 15 more minutes or until the cereal is nicely browned. Add raisins, toasted wheat germ, coconut, or granola.

Extended activities: Think of other foods that are eaten with fingers. Make a chart or a book of "foods that are supposed to be eaten with our hands" and another book or chart of "foods that are supposed to be eaten with a fork or a spoon."

SOYBEAN SUPERSNACKS

 1 *cup rinsed soybeans*
 1½ *cups water*
 1 *teaspoon olive oil*

1. Soak the beans overnight in the refrigerator, drain well, and spread them on a cookie sheet.

2. Bake at 200° F for about 2½ hours, stir with olive oil, and return

to the oven for an additional ½ hour. Store in a tightly covered container.

Extended activities: Hang a piece of chart paper in the science or cooking center. Help the children find pictures of foods that grow in a pod. Cook some other "pod foods."

PICKLED PINK EGGS

Hard-boiled eggs
Beet juice drained from pickled beets

1. Place the eggs in cold water with a pinch of salt. Bring the water to a boil, reduce the heat, and simmer for 15 minutes. Remove and immediately immerse eggs in cold water to make them easier to peel.
2. Let the children crack the eggs all over and roll them gently on the table to loosen the shell.
3. Place the eggs in a jar of pickled beet juice and put them in the refrigerator overnight.
4. When they are pink, serve them with mustard or relish.

Extended activities: Conduct experiments to see what other foods might be used for dyes and what other foods can be dyed with beet juice. (See discussion on food dyes under Visual heading in Chapter 6.)

MISS MUFFET'S FAVORITE SNACK

1 *quart milk*
2 *tablespoons vinegar*
  pineapple or other crushed fruit

1. Heat the milk until bubbles begin to form.
2. Remove from heat, stir in the vinegar, and let the children continue to stir while the mixture cools and curd forms.
3. Separate the curds from the whey by pouring the mixture through a strainer into a glass bowl. Let the children gently press the curds with a wooden spatula to squeeze out the whey.
4. Let the children add fruit to their own serving of curds and stir.

Extended activities: Act out the nursery rhyme, and retell it using the flannel board. Write an experience story detailing what happened when the vinegar was added. Send copies of the story home with the children. Explore other products made from milk. Make butter, for example, or visit a dairy farm.

FRIENDSHIP SOUP

(Individual portions for cup cooking)
vegetables, a variety (have the children bring them in to share with their friends)
meat stock made with bones
alphabet noodles (optional)
hot beverage cups, the paper variety

1. Write the children's names on their cups with a permanent-ink magic marker.
2. Boil the bones until you have a good broth.

3. Let the children wash, peel, cut up the vegetables, and put a small amount of each in their cups.

4. Pour a little broth into each cup, add the noodles.

5. Place the cups in an electric skillet (with about ¾ inch of water in the bottom) and cook on low heat until the vegetables are done.

Extended activities: See Chapter 6 (Biologic Origins of Foods) for other activities using some of the vegetables that were included in this project. Read *Stone Soup*[2] and follow up with activities that promote altruistic behavior. For example, give an award or medal to each child who can think of something "friendly" to do for someone else.

Make a "Friendly Hands Make Happy Hearts" board. For example, each child tells of a friendly action performed by someone else for them. The friendly actions and the children's names are written on strips of paper and decorated by the children. All of the friendly deeds are posted on the board. In the center, display a huge red heart, stuffed by the children with newspaper balls and fringed with children's hand cutouts.

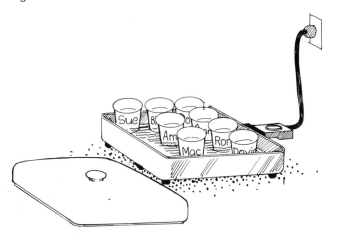

JACK'S SOUP

(Individual portions for cup cooking)

    hot paper cups

1 teaspoon quick-cooking dried beans (or peas)

½ cup cold water

    dash of dried thyme, marjoram, and cayenne

    chopped onion, celery, carrot, and potato

1. Write the children's names on the cups.

2. Preheat the electric skillet to about 350° F. Be sure to cover the bottom of the skillet with about ¾ inch of water first.

3. Let the children chop up each of the vegetables and measure about ½ teaspoonful of each into their cups.

4. Let the children fill their cups one-half full with water from a small

[2]Marcia Brown, *Stone Soup* (New York: Charles Scribner's Sons, 1947).

pitcher if a sink is not available or if it is not low enough for them to reach comfortably.

5. Let the children sprinkle the spices into their cups.

6. When all the cups are ready, place them in the skillet, cover, and let cook for about an hour or until the beans are tender.

7. Variation: If you use peas, add a little milk when the liquid cooks down, heat, and serve.

Extended activities: Read *Jack and the Beanstalk,* sprout some beans, and record their growth. (See sprouting activities under Biologic Origins of Foods in Chapter 6 for additional activities.)

GLAZED CARROT WHEELS

8 carrots

2 tablespoons butter

2 tablespoons honey

½ cup water

1. Let each child scrape ½ carrot and cut into wheels.

2. Melt butter in a large electric skillet.

3. Mix water and honey and pour into the skillet.

4. Add carrots, cover, and cook on low heat, stirring occasionally until tender. Makes about 16 servings.

Extended activities: This is a good "circle" snack, or a snack to reinforce the color orange. Follow-up activities might include art projects on round paper or color mixing to "make" orange. Children could also be encouraged to think of other orange or round foods and to make books to illustrate them. Books can also be made to include the children's favorite carrot recipes. Additional activities include sprouting carrot tops in a jar lid with a little water or planting and growing carrots for a snack. Read *The Carrot Seed.*[3]

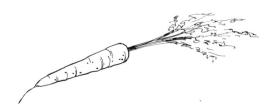

SPICY RICE PUDDING

(Individual portions for cup cooking)

hot paper cups

3 tablespoons brown rice, uncooked

⅛ teaspoon molasses

¼ apple, chopped

dash cinnamon

4 tablespoons milk

a few raisins

[3]Ruth Krauss, *The Carrot Seed* (New York: Scholastic Book Service, 1971).

1. Put the children's names on their cups.

2. Let each child chop a wedge of apple and measure the rice, milk, molasses, and cinnamon into their cups.

3. Place the cups in an electric skillet. The bottom of the skillet should be covered with about ¾ inch water. Cover and cook, stirring frequently until the milk is absorbed.

Extended activities: Examine the raisins before they are cooked. Compare them after they have "plumped." You may wish to use dried apples instead of fresh ones, so that children can see how they can be reconstituted. Follow up by making raisins or by drying apples. See the directions under Food Preparation in Chapter 6.

YOGURT TARTS

½ *pound cottage cheese (You might make your own! See Miss Muffet's Favorite Snack above.)*

1 *cup unsweetened yogurt*
   fresh fruit, one kind or a variety

1 *tablespoon honey*

1 *teaspoon vanilla*

16 *individual tart shells*

1. Let the children chop or slice the fruit and line their shells with it.

2. Whip yogurt, cottage cheese, honey, and vanilla together.

3. Let the children spoon the mixture over their fruit.

4. Refrigerate for an hour before serving.

FOODS FOR CELEBRATIONS

Very young children are rooted in the present; time orientation is difficult for them. Yesterday and tomorrow are two terms they struggle daily to fully understand. When a three-year-old takes a nap, for example, it is not unusual for the child to wake up thinking, "It's tomorrow!" Fours and fives are frequently heard to say, "I went tomorrow" or "I'm going yesterday." Comprehending larger units of time like weeks, months, years, or seasons is even more difficult for them. For this reason, adults need to think of important events with which to mark the passing of time. To capitalize on these events by providing special activities is one way of making seasons memorable to children. Seasonal activities can serve as "time markers."

Cooking activities, because of the intense involvement they stimulate, are especially appropriate time markers. The recipes and cooking experiences in which children participate can be recorded in books or on charts and can be reviewed periodically throughout the year. These records will serve as enjoyable reminders of celebrations shared with friends.

STUFFED APPLES *(Halloween)*

baking apples, cored
any combination of the following: raisins, walnuts, banana slices,

prunes, coconut, orange slices, or pineapple chunks

½ *teaspoon honey per apple*

1. Let each child core an apple.

2. Let children stuff their apples with the ingredients provided. They may need to slice or chop some of the ingredients first.

3. Allow children to dribble the honey over their apple filling.

4. Cover the bottom of a baking dish with hot water, put in the apples, and bake at 400° F for about 45 minutes. While the apples are baking, spoon some of the liquid over them to keep them from drying out. If the children have been allowed to choose from a variety of ingredients for their fillings, each apple will be different and the children won't want them to get "mixed up." A flag made from a toothpick and a folded-over piece of masking tape can be used to identify each child's apple.

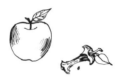

FRESH PUMPKIN THUMBKIN

Thumbkin

½ cup butter	2 eggs
1 tablespoon honey	1¼ cups wheat flour
½ teaspoon molasses	⅓ cup chopped nuts
½ teaspoon vanilla	

1. Let the children chop the nuts.

2. Let the children cream the butter, molasses, and honey.

3. If you have a suitable utensil for separating egg yolks from the whites, let the children do it. Beat and save the egg whites. The children can beat the egg yolk slightly and add it to the butter mixture.

4. Let the children add the vanilla and flour to the mixture and make a dough.

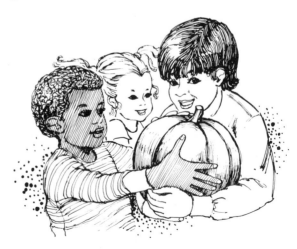

5. Let the children measure the dough (about 1 tablespoon each) and roll it into balls, dip the balls into the egg white, and then roll them in the chopped nuts.

6. Put them on an ungreased cookie sheet and allow each child to mash a thumbprint into each ball to form a little "bowl" for the pumpkin filling.

Pumpkin Filling

pumpkin

pumpkin pie spices or cinnamon and nutmeg

1. To make peeling easier, cut the pumpkin into wedges and place them in a baking dish so that the insides are facing downward. Bake in 250° F oven until the peelings pull off easily.

2. Mash the pumpkin, drain, and mix with spices.

3. Fill the "thumbkins" with the pumpkin, and bake at 375° F for 12 to 15 minutes.

HARVEST MOONS *(Thanksgiving)*

cheddar cheese

salad dressing

1. Soften cheese and moisten slightly with salad dressing.

2. Let the children measure the cheese (about 1 tablespoon each) and roll the cheese into a ball.

INDIAN CORN PUDDING

2 cups drained whole-kernel corn (frozen, fresh, or canned)

½ teaspoon honey

¼ teaspoon pepper

2 eggs

1 cup milk

1 tablespoon margarine

2 tablespoons wheat cracker crumbs

1. Preheat oven to 350° F.

2. Let the children grind the crackers in a metate like the ones the Indians used for grinding grain. You can improvise with a scooped-out stone for a bowl and a small flat rock for pulverizing the crackers.

3. Let the children break and beat the eggs.

4. Let the children measure and mix the ingredients.

5. The children can grease the baking dish (having a capacity of about 1 quart) and pour in the ingredients.

6. Set the dish into a pan with about 1 inch in it and bake for about 70 minutes. Serves about 8.

SWEET POTATO LOAF

2 large sweet potatoes	*2 tablespoons melted margarine*
1 cup whole-wheat flour	*2 eggs*
1 cup cornmeal	*2 tablespoons molasses*
1 teaspoon baking *powder*	*1¼ cups milk*

1. Boil the potatoes until they are tender (about 45 minutes), cool, peel, and let the children dice them.

2. Let the children sift the dry ingredients into a large mixing bowl.

3. Let the children crack and beat the eggs.

4. The children can combine the margarine, eggs, molasses, and milk in another bowl.

5. Let them mix in the dry ingredients and then fold in the sweet potatoes.

6. Pour the batter into two loaf pans and bake at 400° F for an hour.

LATKES *(Chanukah)*

2 *medium potatoes*

1 *egg*

¼ *cup flour*

½ *teaspoon salt*

   applesauce

1. Show the children how to use a potato peeler safely, and let them peel the potatoes.

2. Help the children grate the potatoes coarsely.

3. Let the children break and beat the egg and then mix the potatoes with the egg, flour, and salt.

4. Drop the dough (about 1 tablespoon at a time) into hot vegetable oil and brown on both sides.

5. Serve with applesauce.

CRANBERRY SURPRISE *(Christmas)*

2 *pounds cranberries*

3¾ *cups orange juice*

¼ *cup honey*

4 *tablespoons plain gelatin*

2 *orange rinds, grated*

2 *16¼-ounce cans crushed pineapple*

2 *cups walnuts*

1 *pint whipping cream*

1. Let the children wash the cranberries and then boil them in the orange juice until they pop. Add the honey and gelatin.

2. The children can chop the walnuts, grate the orange rind, and help to beat the whipping cream while the cranberry mixture cools.

3. Add the orange rind, pineapple, and walnuts.

4. Gently fold the whipped cream into the mixture, pour into molds (Christmas symbol molds, perhaps), and refrigerate. Serves about 16.

CHILDREN-OF-THE-WORLD FROSTIE[4] *(Martin Luther King's Birthday)*

Strawberries (red)

Pineapple, crushed or fresh (yellow)

Black cherries (black)

White pears (white)

[4]The colors in the Frostie represent the races referred to in the song, "Jesus Loves the Little Children."

¼ *cup fruit juice or ginger ale per child*

1. Let the children wash and finely chop the fruit.

2. Pour the fruit into ice cube trays and freeze. (It may be necessary to stir in a little fruit juice first.)

3. Let each of the children pour ¼ cup fruit juice (perhaps pineapple) and ¼ cup ginger ale into their cups and add a fruit cube or two apiece.

COLD HEARTS *(Valentine's Day)*

8 tablespoons unflavored gelatin

4 cups cranberry juice

1. Let the children measure and mix the gelatin with ½ cup juice.

2. Boil another ½ cup juice and add to the gelatin mixture. Stir to dissolve. Add the remaining 3 cups juice and stir.

3. Pour into two 9-inch pans and chill until firm.

4. Use a valentine cookie cutter to cut into hearts.

5. Eat with fingers.

6. The leftover trimmings can be saved and mixed with yogurt for another snack.

HAMENTASCHEN (HAMEN'S POCKET) *(Purim)*

1 package yellow cake mix

1 cup flour

2 eggs

2 tablespoons water

1. Preheat oven to 365°F.

2. Let the children combine all of the ingredients in a large bowl and mix well.

3. Give each child a small amount (approximately 2 tablespoons) of dough and let them roll their dough onto a floured surface to about 2½ to 3 inches in size.

4. Let them prick their dough and measure about 1 teaspoon of prune filling (or fruit or jam) into the center.

5. To make Hamen's pocket (a pocket for the fruit), the children should "pinch up" three corners.

6. Bake for 6 minutes.

SPICY TREASURE *(Columbus Day)*

½ *cup butter*	¼ *teaspoon ginger*
¾ *cup molasses*	¼ *teaspoon cloves*
3 eggs	½ *teaspoon allspice*
1 cup buttermilk	*1½ teaspoons cinnamon*
2 cups whole-wheat flour	*1 teaspoon baking soda*

1. Let the children cream the butter and molasses.

2. The children can crack and beat the eggs and then add them to the butter and molasses.

3. Place a sifter in a bowl and measure all the dry ingredients into it.

4. In a large bowl, add the rest of the ingredients, alternating first a

little of the wet ingredients and then a little of the dry. Mix well each time until all the ingredients are mixed.

5. Let the children grease a cake pan 9 by 13 inches in size, and pour the batter in.

6. Bake at 375° F for about 30 minutes.

CHERRY TARTS *(George Washington's Birthday)*

Use the Thumbkin pastry for the tart (see recipe for Fresh Pumpkin Thumbkin above). Fill with cherry pie filling.

LINCOLN LOG SNACKS *(Lincoln's Birthday)*

See the Lincoln Log recipe illustrated in the Individual Portion, No-Cook Snacks section of this chapter.

SAINT PATRICK'S DAY TREAT

Make Pretzel Initials (see recipe above) into snakes like the ones Saint Patrick drove from Ireland, or make shamrock finger jello using the Cold Hearts recipe above, substituting limeade for the liquid.

EGGS IN NESTS *(Easter)*

1   can Chinese noodles
1   cup mayonnaise
2   grated carrots
1   cup small seedless grapes
    a small, unused meat tray for each child

1. Let the children wash, peel, and grate the carrots.

2. Let the children mix the mayonnaise, noodles, and carrots in a large bowl. You may have to increase the amount of mayonnaise to get the noodles to stick together to form a nest.

3. Let each child arrange a scoop of noodles on their trays and add a few eggs (grapes).

4. Refrigerate for 1 hour.

CHAROSET *(Passover)*

5   apples
½   cup grape juice
1   cup walnuts
     cinnamon to taste

1. Let the children wash, core, and chop the apples.

2. The children should shell the walnuts into the measuring cup so they can determine when they have a full measure. Predicting how many more will be needed to fill the cup is an important part of this task. When the cup is filled, they can chop the walnuts.

3. Let the children mix the apples, nuts, and grape juice into a large bowl.

4. Place some cinnamon on a napkin for the children to smell and taste before sprinkling it into the mixture. You may also want to let them examine a cinnamon stick.

5. Stir. Then, let the children measure about 2 tablespoons of the treat into their cups. Enjoy!

MAY FLOWERS *(Mayday)*

Some flowers are for eating! Cauliflowers, for example, and Brussels sprouts. Eat them raw, with a dip, or make flower pops by freezing them.

INDEPENDENCE ICE CREAM SNACK *(Independence Day)*

Exert your independence by choosing your own ice cream topping.

1 14-ounce can of Eagle Brand Condesed Milk
2 tablespoons water
2 egg yolks
4 teaspoons vanilla
1 pint whipping cream

1. Let children help to separate the egg yolks and beat them.

2. Let the children help to whip the cream. If the beater is loud, warn them before turning it on. Let them take turns helping to hold the beater (if it is the hand-held variety).

3. Combine all ingredients except the whipped cream in a large bowl. Then fold in the whipped cream, pour into a foil-lined loaf pan 9 by 5 inches in size, and freeze until firm (about 6 hours).

4. Serve with a choice of toppings like wheat germ, crushed nuts, carob sauce, pineapple, bananas, or other fresh fruits which the children have helped to prepare.

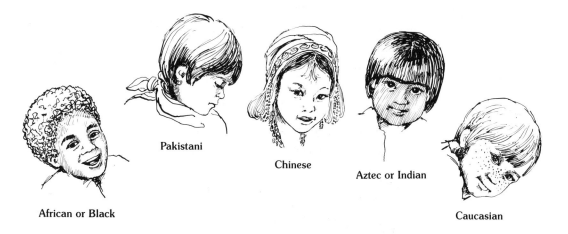

Pakistani

Chinese

Aztec or Indian

African or Black

Caucasian

FOODS FROM MANY CULTURES

An effort should always be made to prepare foods that are familiar to the cultural groups that are represented by the children in your program. It is one way of promoting a sense of security in the child and of building a closer relationship with their families. Preparing foods from cultures that are unfamiliar to the children in your group is also beneficial to help expand their awareness that the world is a home for many different peoples and races. Favorite "soul foods," for instance, should be introduced in ways that not only promote acceptance of differing cuisines but respect for the ideas and preferences of others. In Chapter 3, some ideas for integrating ethnic foods with representative art and music activities are described. Activities like these can serve to heighten the children's awareness of the special contributions that have been made by various cultural groups.

TAMALE CASSEROLE

2 onions	2 teaspoons chili powder
1 pound ground beef	3 cups cornmeal
2 16-ounce cans tomatoes	4 eggs
2 16½-ounce cans creamed corn	2 cups milk
2 9-ounce cans pitted black olives	

1. Let children peel and chop onions. Sauté chopped onion in oil.
2. Let children measure and mix beef, onions, tomatoes, corn, olives, and chili powder.
3. Let children break and mix eggs and combine with milk and cornmeal.
4. Let children combine both mixtures and bake in casserole at 350°F for one hour.

MEXICAN SKILLET BREAD

1 cup cooked kidney beans	2 teaspoons chili powder
1½ cups water	1 teaspoon cumin
2 onions	⅔ cup cheddar cheese
2 eggs	2 teaspoons baking powder
2 cups cornmeal	

1. Let the children peel and chop the onions. Sauté them in a large, heavy skillet (or two small ones).
2. Let the children help grate the cheese.
3. In a large bowl, mix all the other ingredients, except the cheese and onions, pour the mixture into the skillet, mix, and let the children sprinkle the cheese on top.
4. Bake at 350° F for about 20 minutes.

GAZPACHO

6 cups tomato juice	½ teaspoon dill weed
4 fresh tomatoes or 1 16-ounce can of pared tomatoes	2 tablespoons olive oil
1 cucumber	1 onion
juice of 1 lemon	½ green pepper
½ teaspoon tarragon	2½ tablespoons wine vinegar
½ teaspoon basil	⅓ cup fresh or 1 teaspoons dried parsley

1. Let the children peel and chop the onion into fine pieces. Then chop the parsley, bell pepper, and tomatoes. (If canned tomatoes are used, drain them first.)

2. Show the children how to use a peeler to remove some of the peeling from the cucumber. It should be "stripped." Then the children can dice it.

3. Let the children measure the spices, oil, vinegar, and tomato juice, and mix them with the chopped vegetables.

4. Chill for an hour or more.

GUACAMOLE

1 ripe avocado

½ onion

1 teaspoon lemon juice

1 ripe tomato

¼ cup mayonnaise

1. Remove the pit from the avocado and save it to sprout.

2. Peel the avocado, and let the children mash it. The children can finely chop the tomato and onion.

3. Combine all the ingredients and serve as a dip.

NEW ORLEANS POTATO SALAD

9 cold boiled potatoes	*¾ cup salad dressing*
3 spring onions	*3 hard-boiled eggs*
2 celery stalks	*2 green peppers*
½ teaspoon black pepper	*juice of ½ lemon or lime*

1. Let the children chop the potatoes, onions, eggs, and celery.

2. Let the children squeeze the lemon and remove the seeds from the juice to save for sprouting.

3. Mix all the ingredients in a large bowl and chill for a few hours.

BORSCHT

1½ tablespoons soft margarine	*5 cups combination vegetable stock and water*
5 onions	
5 potatoes	*½ teaspoon dill weed*
1½ cups beets	*5 teaspoons cider vinegar*
2 stalks celery	*4 teaspoons honey*
4½ cups cabbage	*1½ cups tomato puree*
1 teaspoon caraway seeds	*1 cup plain yogurt*

1. Simmer potatoes and beets until tender. Save the water.

2. Let the children chop the celery and cabbage and thinly slice the potatoes and beets.

3. Let the children chop the onions and help to sauté them with margarine and caraway seeds. When the onions are transparent, add the celery and cabbage, then the stock from the water and potatoes, and finally all the other ingredients except the yogurt. Cook until the vegetables are tender.

4. When you are ready to serve, mix ⅔ cup yogurt with the borscht and use the rest of the yogurt for a garnish.

KUGEL

3 eggs	1½ cups cottage cheese
1¾ cups plain yogurt	½ teaspoon vanilla
2 teaspoons cinnamon	2 tablespoons honey
2 baking apples	4 cups wide, flat egg noodles

1. Boil noodles until they are just tender. Do not overcook.

2. Let the children slice the apples and break and lightly beat the eggs.

3. Help the children measure the remaining ingredients into a bowl and mix with apples and eggs.

4. The children can butter a casserole dish (9 by 13 inches) while they wait for the noodles to cook.

5. Pour the mixture into the dish, sprinkle with bread crumbs, and bake uncovered for 40 minutes at 375° F.

MINESTRONE

2 cups cooked chickpeas (save stock)	⅓ cup raisins
	1 turnip
3 onions	2 cups green peas
1 teaspoon olive oil	1 cup whole-wheat noodles
1 teaspoon oregano	3 carrots
1 teaspoon dried basil	2 cups green beans
dash of cinnamon and ground black pepper	½ head cabbage
	1 teaspoon red wine vinegar
8 fresh or 1 large can tomatoes	

1. Let the children chop the onions and sauté them in olive oil with oregano, basil, cinnamon, and black pepper.

2. Let the children chop the tomatoes and stir them with their juice into the onions. Let this mixture simmer while you prepare the other vegetables.

3. Let the children chop the carrots and turnips and add to the soup. Simmer for about 30 minutes. Add the green beans and cook for an additional 20 minutes.

4. Add the chickpeas and their broth, the peas, cabbage, noodles, wine vinegar, and any water that is needed for desired thickness.

5. When the last vegetables are tender, serve with sprinkles of Parmesan, ricotta, or cottage cheese.

RIESKA

2 cups whole-wheat flour

1 teaspoon sugar

1 cup undiluted evaporated milk

2 teaspoons baking powder

1 tablespoon margarine

1. Melt the butter and combine with milk.

2. Let the children measure and combine all the other ingredients and then stir in the milk and butter.

3. Stir until a smooth dough forms, and turn out onto an oiled cookie sheet.

4. Let the children dip their hands into flour to dust them lightly, and pat the dough out into a 15-inch circle about ½ inch in thickness.

5. Prick the dough with a fork all over and bake at 450° F for about 10 minutes. Serve hot with butter.

LEBANESE SALAD

½ cooked chickpeas	2 cucumbers
3 cups bulgur	4 tomatoes
6 cups boiling water	juice of 1 lemon
3 cups chopped parsley	½ cup olive oil
½ cup chopped onions	spinach or cabbage,
4 teaspoons dried mint	shredded

1. Soak the bulgur in hot water until the wheat is fluffy (about 15 minutes). Drain and press excess water out through the strainer.

2. Let the children chop the parsley, onions, tomatoes, and cucumbers.

3. Mix all ingredients and chill. Serve with garnish of mint or sprouts.

HUMMUS

1 cup canned chickpeas

¼ cup sesame-seed butter

1 tablespoon olive oil

  juice of 2 lemons

2 tablespoons fresh parsley

1. Let the children squeeze lemons and chop parsley.

2. Measure all ingredients into a blender and blend until smooth.

SUKIYAKI

1 pound round steak, cut in thin strips	1 teaspoon soy sauce
	1 8-ounce can bamboo shoots
½ cup mushrooms	3 tablespoons water
4 spring onions	3 cups raw spinach leaves
2 stalks celery	3 cups cooked brown rice
2 onions	

1. Brown the steak in a wok or non-stick frying pan.

2. Let the children cut the spring onions (including the stems) lengthwise.

3. Let the children wash and chop the celery, mushrooms, onions, and spinach leaves.

4. Stir all the ingredients except the spinach and rice into the wok. When the vegetables are tender, add the spinach and stir until it wilts.

5. Serve over rice.

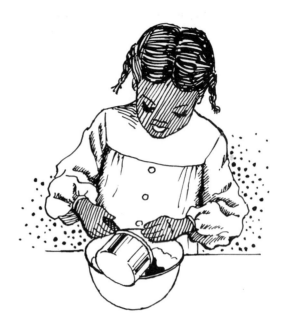

WON-TON SOUP

½ *pound lean ground pork*　　2 *teaspoons cornstarch*
2 *spring onions*　　　　　　　1 *tablespoon water*
8 *water chestnuts*　　　　　　1 *package won-ton skins*
1 *tablespoon light soy sauce*　½ *cup chicken broth per child*
¼ *teaspoon ground ginger*

1. Let children chop onions and chestnuts.

2. Combine all ingredients in a large bowl. Mix well.

3. Place 1 teaspoon mixture into the center of each won-ton skin, fold over, and stick edges together. You may have to dampen the edges slightly with water. Pinch around the meat to seal it in. Then pull the bottom corners together and pinch firmly to seal (like a fortune cookie). Use a little water if necessary. Be careful not to let the won ton dry out while the children are working. It may be necessary to cover them with a damp cloth as they are folded.

4. Add the won ton to boiling water, return to boil, add a cup of cold water, and allow the water to return to a boil.

5. Heat the chicken broth and drop a won ton or two in each child's soup as it is served.

FRIED RICE

2 *eggs*
2 *spring onions*
½ *cup cooked diced pork or chicken*
4 *cups cooked brown rice*
3 *tablespoons soy sauce*
2 *tablespoons peanut oil*

122

1. Let the children crack and scramble the eggs. Set them aside.

2. Let the children dice the onions and meat and stir-fry them until they are heated through. Set them aside and heat the rice with two tablespoons oil.

3. Combine all ingredients and stir until they are thoroughly heated and evenly distributed.

VIETNAMESE SPINACH SOUP

8 cups chicken broth

1 pound frozen spinach

1 cup cooked brown rice

Bring the broth to a boil and add rice and then spinach. Cook only until tender.

NIGERIAN SOUP

1 cup cooked chicken, diced	*1 onion*
1 cup chicken broth	*1 cup roasted peanuts*
1 beef bouillon	*½ cup milk*
1 tomato	*3 tablespoons rice*
1 potato	

1. Let children wash and dice potato, tomato, and onion. Simmer for 30 minutes in broth and bouillon.

2. Let the children shell and roast the peanuts, and drop them into the blender with the milk. Chop until they are fine but still crunchy.

3. Combine the peanut mixture with the rice and add to the soup. Simmer for about 30 more minutes.

REVIEW ACTIVITIES

1. Choose a recipe from this chapter. Make a picture recipe.

2. Review the goals given in the list at the beginning of this chapter and list the possibilities for learning. Write your goals and the cooking activity in lesson plan form (see Table 5-1).

   a. Look for some related activities in Chapter 6 to add to your lesson plan.

   b. Complete the activities with the children.

   c. Record the children's comments during the activity. What do you think they learned? Were they able to follow the recipe chart, or should the chart be altered or changed to make it more readable the next time?

3. Begin a collection of celebration recipes. Share them with others who work with children.

4. Write a letter to the parents explaining the value of cooking with children. Use some ideas from the list of goals.

BAXTER, KATHLEEN (Illus.), *Come and Get It: A Natural Foods Cookbook for Children.* Ann Arbor, Mich.: Children First Press, 1981.

BRUNO, J., and P. DAKAN, *Cooking in the Classroom.* Belmont, Calif.: Fearon Publishers, Inc., 1974.

COBB, VICKI, *Arts and Crafts You Can Eat.* New York: Harper & Row Publishers, Inc. 1974.

COHL, VICKI, *Science Experiments You Can Eat.* Philadelphia: J.B. Lippincott Company, 1973.

COOPER, JANE, *Love at First Bite,* New York: Alfred A. Knopf, Inc., 1977.

COOPER, TERRY TOUF, and MARILYN RATNER, *Many Hands Cooking: An International Cookbook for Boys and Girls.* New York: Harper & Row Publishers, Inc. 1974.

CROFT, KAREN B., *The Good For Me Cookbook.* Palo Alto, Calif.: R & E Research Associates, 1971.

———— ,*The Taming of the Cookie Monster.* Wayzata, Minn.: Meadowbrook Press, 1977.

FERREIRA, NANCY, *Learning through Cooking: A Cooking Program for Children from Two to Ten.* Palo Alto, Calif.: R & E Research Associates, 1982.

FERREIRA, NANCY, "Teacher's Guide to Educational Cooking in the Nursery School." *Young Children,* November 1973.

FRIEDLANDER, BARBARA, *Cookbook for the New Age: Earth, Water, Fire, Air.* New York: Macmillan, Inc., 1972.

GOODWIN, MARY T., and GERRY POLLEN, *Creative Food Experiences for Children.* Washington, D.C.: Center for Science in the Public Interest, 1974.

JOHNSON, BARBARA, and BETTY PLEMONS, *Cup Cooking.* Lake Alfred, Fla.: Early Education Press, 1978.

KAPLAN, LISA, *Once Upon a Cook Book.* Palo Alto, Calif.: Good Sign Publications, 1981.

LANSKY, VICKI, *Feed Me, I'm Yours.* Wayzata, Minn.: Meadowbrook Press, 1974.

MARBACK, ELLEN, PLASS, MARTHA and LILLY HSU O'CONNELL, *Nutrition in a Changing World.* Provo, Utah: Brigham Young Univ. Press, 1983.

MCAFEE, ORALIE, EVELYN HAINES, and BARBARA YOUNG, *Cooking and Eating with Children.* Washington, D.C.: Association for Childhood Education International, 1974.

MCCLENAHAN, PAT, and IDA JAQUE, *Cool Cooking for Kids.* Belmont, Calif.: Fearon Publishers, Inc., 1976.

Parents' Nursery School, *Kids Are Natural Cooks.* Cambridge, Mass.

PAUL, AILEEN, *Kids Cooking without a Stove,* New York: Doubleday and Company Inc., 1975.

WARNER, PENNY, *Healthy Snacks for Kids,* Concord Calif: Nitty Gritty Productions, 1983.

WARREN, JEAN, *Super Snacks,* Alderwood Manner, WA: Warren Publishing House, 1982.

WHITENER, CAROLE, *Snacks to Grow On.* Chesapeake, Va., 1982.

chapter six

nutrition **ACTIVITIES**
for young children

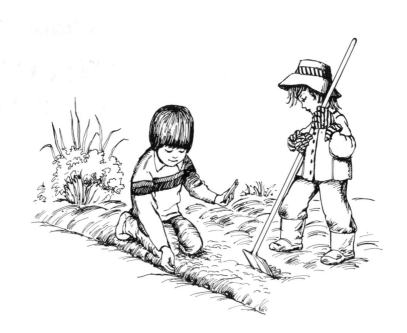

OBJECTIVES

After reading this chapter the reader will be able to:

- Plan creative food experiences that are appropriate for preschool children.
- Provide experiences that are prerequisites for the formation of advanced abstract nutrition concepts.

Young children learn through sensory exploration; poking, smearing, smelling, tasting, and squishing are some of their natural learning behaviors. For this reason, children must have hands-on experiences with real food objects to develop new concepts about food. The popular practice of teaching young children nutrition with work sheets and food pictures is less effective than first-hand experience because of the limited information that pictures can provide. For example, little that is new can be learned about radishes by looking at a picture of a radish. The information not presented in the picture must be furnished by images produced in the mind of the child. But if the child's experiences with radishes are limited, the images will be incomplete, for they will lack the cues that are necessary for the recall of smell, taste, texture, contents, origin, weight, and size.

A more appropriate approach for teaching young children about food is to involve them in growing it, cutting it, sorting it into groups by size, making comparisons in weight and color, and smelling and eating it.

There are no shortcuts to familiarizing children with various foods. Following experiences with foods, however, the technique of using pictures to represent foods that have already been explored by the children can be effective.

The following episode related to the authors by a kindergarten teacher provides an illustration.

The class of five-year-olds planted their spring garden in the schoolyard with radishes, corn, squash, and watermelons. Each day they tended the garden, pulling weeds, watering, checking for insects, and watching the plants grow. In the classroom while they waited for the plants to mature and bear fruit, they watched films of food in various stages of growth and arranged "plant-part" pieces on flannel boards to show that they had learned facts such as which vegetables grow under the ground and which vegetables grow on vines and stalks.

After what seemed to be an interminable wait, the first vegetables—radishes—were ready for the harvest! The children eagerly began to pull them up. "You can see the red part sticking out of the dirt," they squealed excitedly. Some of the children began digging around the base of the other vegetables in the garden. "How will we know when the corn is ready to pull up?" they asked. "Will the watermelons stick out of the dirt?" they asked as they scraped the dirt away from the stems on the watermelon vines.

The teacher, feeling perplexed, answered, "Don't you remember the films that we saw of watermelons growing on *vines*?"

"Yes, but how will we know when to pull them up?" they asked, ignoring her cue. She tried to remind them of the many activities they had done in the classroom while they waited for the garden to grow—games like vegetable and fruit lotto, sorting games, and the flannel board station—all designed to teach them how vegetables in their garden would grow. The children continued to investigate the stems of all of the vegetables, convinced that they would discover parts of other vegetables sticking out from the soil at the base of their stalks.

The manner in which young children think is a constant source of amazement to adults. Quite possibly, if this teacher had not planted the garden, but had instead relied on classroom teaching aids to help her explain food origins, she may never have known that even though the children were able to manipulate the flannel board pieces and give correct rote responses to her questions, they did not really "understand" the food facts presented. In this case, the learning behavior of the children in the classroom was misleading to the teacher.

Children younger than six or seven, in addition to having limited representational abilities and requiring first-hand experience for concept formation, exhibit many other unique characteristics that make the practice of "watering down" upper-level curriculum inappropriate. One example that has a bearing on how nutrition education should be structured in programs for young children is found by examining the classification abilities of young children. Preoperational children, that is, children between the ages of two and six or seven, according to Piaget (1964), are able to classify on the basis of only one property at a time. Therefore, the task of separating green vegetables from red vegetables, especially if other foods that are not vegetables are included in the master group, would be too difficult for most five-year-olds. For this reason, the traditional approach in which the four food groups provide the structure for nutrition activities may be less appropriate for these children.

Some of the prerequisite nutritional concepts to the advanced abstract ideas in many nutrition education guides are presented in this chapter. They are presented in four sections: (1) Food Properties, (2) Our Bodies Need Food, (3) Biologic Origins of Foods, and (4) Food Preparation. Each section is accompanied by activities for preoperational children and provides numerous opportunities for integrating nutritional education with other areas of the early childhood curriculum.

FOOD PROPERTIES

As previously mentioned, familiarity with a food helps to ensure its acceptance. To become familiar with a food, however, requires that it be fully explored. Each new food discovery gained by eating, pouring, mixing, or otherwise manipulating the food will add to the child's "file" of knowledge about foods in general. As the "file" grows larger and more diverse, it will become necessary for the child to organize newly acquired knowledge into categories and to begin to compare new foods with previously discovered foods. This marks the beginning of the ability to classify and lays the foundation for later understandings of food grouping.

The first nutritional experiences should, perhaps, be designed to focus the attention of each of the senses on the unique properties of each food that is presented. The child's perceptions can then be discussed and perhaps recorded on charts or in a child-made book like the one shown in Figure 6-1. If this technique is used, it is important, following the completion of sensorial activities, to encourage the child or the group to dictate their impressions to the adult. The adult prints the words of the children into the book exactly as they are spoken. These can be kept as lasting mementoes of the experience and read later to parents or friends. This practice has many benefits, as follows:

1. It sharpens the observation skills of the children.

2. It encourages children to notice similarities and differences in color, texture, smell, quantity, and quality and the ways in which foods react to force (cutting, mashing, and rolling), changes in temperature (freezing, cooking, and melting), and the passing of time (aging process).

3. It encourages children to use mathematical and scientific terminology in their descriptions of measurement, space, and changes in matter.

4. It requires that children verbalize their observations; verbalizing helps to clarify and refine the concepts formed during the activities and to expand the vocabularies of children.

5. It teaches children that events and information can be recorded on paper in symbolic form (such as a child-made recipe or a menu), and reviewed or used at a later time by themselves or by others.

An example of how this technique can be used with children as a culminating activity follows. The objective stated at the beginning of the lesson describes the behavior that is to be exhibited by at least 80 percent of the children after all of the activities are completed. Bookmaking is the last activity that is presented in this sequence.

OBJECTIVE

The child will sort pictures of foods that are sweet into one group and pictures of foods that taste salty into another group.

FIGURE 6-1

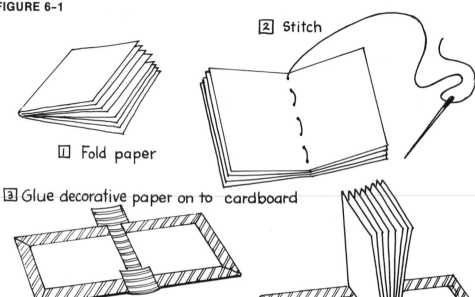

2 Stitch

1 Fold paper

3 Glue decorative paper on to cardboard

4 Glue strip for back

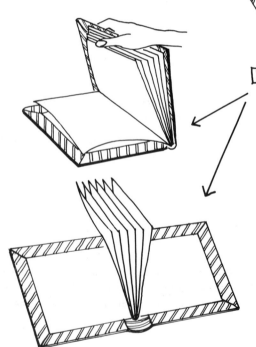

5 Glue front and back pages on to boards.

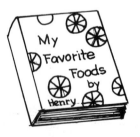

My Favorite Foods by Henry

6 Give your book a title. (Don't forget the by line!)

132

PROCEDURE

This sequence of activities should be completed by individuals or small groups of children over a period of several days, with each activity lasting for 7 to 10 minutes.

1. Use an empty puzzle tray or a box top as a tracing tray (or make individual ones with wide-mouth mayonnaise jar lids). Allow the children to spread a thin layer of salt on the bottom. Children will use the salt tray to trace pictures and doodle designs with their fingers. Tasting should be encouraged but not stressed. Use the salt in the tray for a few days and then repeat the activity using sugar instead of salt.

2. Fill small individual cups one-half full of water. Ask the children to taste the water and to discuss the taste. Sift some salt into the water and stir. Ask, Where did the salt go? Allow the children to taste again. Explore the idea that the salt "dissolved" and that, even though it cannot be seen, it can still be tasted. Repeat the activity with sugar. Discuss some other things that dissolve in liquids. Provide children with other ingredients similar in appearance (flour, corn starch, baking powder).

3. Put salt and sugar in separate containers and give them to the children to examine. Help them to make a book to record their perceptions of the similarities and differences.

BOOK

Page 1. (Draw a symbol for an eye.) Divide the page in half. On one side, record the words that the children use to describe the appearance of salt, and on the other side, the appearance of sugar. Encourage them to use a magnifying glass to examine each more closely and to compare the size of the grains. Ask questions like: Can you think of some other things that look like salt or like sugar?

Page 2. (Draw a symbol for a nose.) Explore and record findings. Put salt and sugar in separate opaque containers with holes in the tops. Ask, Can you smell the difference? Do they have distinctive odors?

Page 3. (Draw a symbol for an ear.) Play a listening game. Ask questions like, When you shake salt (or sugar) in a bottle, does it make a loud sound, a soft sound, or no sound? What else could make that sound? If you bite it, will it crunch? A loud crunch? (Be sure to record their responses in full sentences, preferably in their own words on each sheet of their book.)

Page 4. (Draw a symbol for a finger.) Compare textures. Ask, How did they feel in the tracing tray? Rough? Smooth? Rub some of each between your fingers. Can you think of some other things that feel like salt or sugar? (List them.)

Page 5. (Draw a symbol for a mouth.) Compare tastes. Ask, Can you think of some foods that each taste reminds you of? (Record responses.)

Page 6. (Draw a symbol for a salt box.) Have pictures of sweet and salty foods ready for pasting onto this page. Use pictures of foods that have been recently tasted by the children, examples include potato chips, bacon, raisins, pineapple chunks, and cookies. Variation: Children suggest foods, adult (or child) illustrates as the adult labels the food symbols.

Page 7. (Draw a symbol for a box of sugar.) Children paste or draw pictures of sweet foods on this page.

Below are some additional activities to promote sensorial exploration of food properties. These activities will provide for visual, olfactory, auditory, and tactile exploration.

Visual

Food grouping. Provide as many of the different varieties of the same food as possible, for example, beans (navy, pinto), apples (red, yellow, green), and onions (Spanish, spring). Encourage the children to group them by size, shape, weight, and in as many other ways as can be found. Make books to record the findings. Some examples for book titles to extend this activity are

1. My Book of Big (or Small) Vegetables
2. My Book of Red (Green, Yellow, and so forth) Foods
3. My Book of Long (Round, Pear-Shaped) Foods
4. What Does It Look Like on the Outside? (A book for grouping foods according to their outer coverings, for example, shells [shrimp, eggs, nuts], skins [onions, chicken], peelings [oranges, apples], husks [corn, rice, wheat].)

Food printing. Butterfish make attractive prints. Brush black tempera or printer's ink onto the fish, and press the fish onto paper. The children will delight in seeing the impression made by the outline of the fish eyes, scales, and fins. Vegetables and fruits are also good for printing. Cut the vegetables or fruit in halves and dip them into a shallow pan of thickly mixed tempera. Press them onto the paper to make an impression. Since young children will usually try to scrub or paint with them, they should be shown how to "walk" the food across the paper to make "tracks." Their finished work can be cut into the shape of the vegetable or fruit that was used for printing and mounted on a solid paper of the appropriate color. The background paper should also be cut into the shape of the food.

Food dyes. Make dyes from foods. Boil Spanish onion skins, beets, spinach, or pine needles to make dyes. Dip-dye absorbent, folded paper, fabrics, or natural fiber yarns into the dyes. Use the papers and fabrics for book covers and the yarn for weavings or collages.

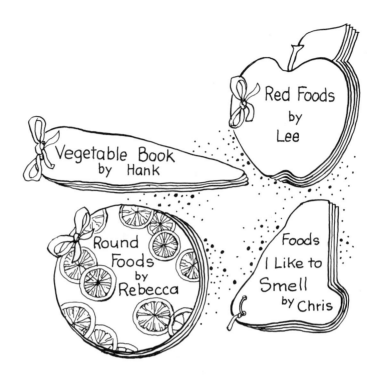

Food collages. Save egg shells, peelings, hulls, husks, and corn silks to use in collages and other art projects. A meat tray can provide a nice backing for a blob of spackeling compound into which dyed noodles, seeds, and other throw-away food materials can be submerged.

Noodle necklaces. Make large noodle necklaces with macaroni. Dye the macaroni by dipping it briefly into food coloring mixed with warm water and a little vinegar. Do not allow the macaroni to stay in the water long enough to soften. String the macaroni on heavy yarn which has had one end stiffened with tape.

Color salads. Make a color salad for snacktime. For example, a green salad might include every imaginable kind of food that is green. Challenge the children to bring green foods from home to add to the salad. On another day change the color. Record the recipe, using the techniques illustrated in Chapter 5. Copy the recipe and share it with friends.

Olfactory

Smelly cans. Make smelly cans from opaque containers with holes in the tops. Put food for smelling in each container. Children are to match the smell to the picture of the food that gives that smell. Be sure to make the activity self-correcting by coding the back of each card to match a code

135

on the bottom of each of the corresponding containers. Some examples of foods to explore are celery, onion, lemon, apple, banana, and pineapple. Include some recently explored "new" foods like mangoes or avacados or flavorings like vanilla or vinegar.

Sniff and tell. Place items (red, yellow, and green apples) in separate brown sandwich bags. Punch a small hole in the side of each bag. Children are to smell each bag and guess the contents. Ask them to decide if they can discriminate between the red apples and the green and yellow apples by smelling them. Try this activity with a variety of fruits and vegetables.

Pudding paintings. Mix instant pudding with water instead of milk, using a little less liquid than the directions call for. The children are to finger-paint on slick paper with the pudding (2 tablespoons per child). Some interesting pudding smells to explore are banana, strawberry, avocado, butterscotch, and chocolate. Add some food coloring to brighten the color if necessary.

Strawberry smacks. Use the recipe for pudding painting described above. Place a spoonful of strawberry pudding on each child's piece of waxed paper (about 5 by 5 inches). Encourage the children to first put their lips into the pudding and then to "kiss" their paper (which can be cut into the shape of a heart). Chin and nose prints will also become instruments for printing!

Sniff books. Paste a piece of fine sandpaper on separate pages of a blank, child-made book. Rub each paper with a different spice. Record children's descriptions of each smell. For example, smells like pumpkin pie. This is a good activity to use on Columbus Day since Columbus was looking for spices on his voyage.

Scratch-and-sniff paintings. Add orange, lemon, banana, or vanilla extract to the appropriate color of liquid tempera paint. Allow the children to paint with these mixtures for several days. Encourage them to smell their work.

Smell dough. Add extracts to a home-made salt dough of the appropriate color.

Sniff pillows. Cut two large circles from sturdy paper (butcher paper or paper bags) to make a giant orange. Staple the circles together, leaving an opening on one side. The children are to wad strips of newspaper and "stuff" the circle until it is full. Staple it closed, and allow the children to paint it on both sides with the orange-scented paint. (Be sure to mix a little liquid starch with the paint to prevent popping and flaking.) Repeat this activity using other food shapes and colors.

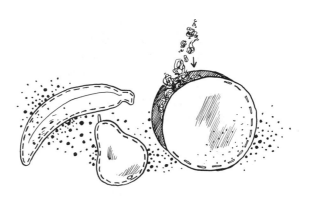

Auditory

Crunchy book. Make a book of foods that crunch when eaten. Children should illustrate and dictate the contents of the book. Decorate the cover with celery prints (technique described in the Visual section above). Variations: Make books of crisp foods, of foods that can squish or slosh, or of quiet foods.

Shake-and-listen cans. Put three kinds of dry food grossly varied in size, such as flour, rice, and beans, into separate opaque plastic containers. Children can shake and match the containers with cards that have samples of these foods glued on them. Variation: Make two sets of containers and let the children match "like" sounds. Occasionally, replace these foods with others to renew interest in the activity. Record the words used to describe these sounds on a chart.

Tactile

Texture paint. Add grits, oatmeal, cornmeal, or other granular foods to home-made finger paint. The recipe for finger paint below is easy to make the very inexpensive. It can be made without color ahead of time. Then the children can use salt shakers to sift powdered tempera paint in colors of their choice onto their paper and work it into the paint. The children can also sprinkle ingredients for textural exploration directly into their paint.

FINGER PAINT RECIPE

Mix 1 cup cornstarch and 2 tablespoons of dry tempera with two quarts of water. Cook, while stirring steadily, until the mixture reaches the desired consistency. Then, add ¼ cup of Ivory Snow detergent and stir. This makes enough for about 25 finger paintings.

Tracing tray. Vary the ingredients in the tracing trays described in the first section of this chapter; try oatmeal, flour, or cornstarch for starters. Then try some brown ingredients like spices and brown sugar. Grouping ingredients that are in some way similar allows children to observe their simi-

137

larities while also focusing attention on their differences. Ways in which ingredients are similar or different can be discussed and the children's words to describe them can be recorded on a chart. Little "baggies" with samples can be mounted on the chart beside their descriptions for future reference.

Feely tubs. Place recycled margarine tubs inside discarded socks. Put fruits, vegetables, nuts, and other familiar foods in them. Let the children feel and guess the contents of each tub. You might also provide pictures of these foods on cards. The pictures can be matched with the tubs that contain the pictured foods.

Taste

Tasty books. Make tasty books in which children illustrate foods that are tart, peppery, tangy, and so forth. Encourage and introduce descriptive terminology.

Snack making. Because children do not trust "blind" taste tests, most tasting experiences should be in coordination with food preparation activities, like cooking or snack making. These are described in detail in Chapters 4 and 5.

OUR BODIES NEED FOOD

It is difficult for adults to teach children that food that tastes good is not always good for their bodies. Just as children at the preoperational stage of development have limited classification abilities, they are also often unable to understand cause and effect relationships and to attend to transformations in events and objects. They are ruled by their own perceptions; the way things *appear* to them is the way things *are*. Efforts to persuade them differently meet with only limited success. To illustrate, most adults have had the experience of trying to divide some juice between two children when two glasses of the same size were not available. The typical five-year-old cannot be convinced that her short, fat glass, filled to the brim can contain as much juice as her sibling's half-filled, tall, skinny glass, if the level of liquid in her glass is lower than that in her sibling's. Even after repeated efforts to teach children that the volume remains the same but has merely taken the shape of the container, preoperational children remain unconvinced. They are ruled by the way things look to them. Likewise, the egocentric thinking of the preoperational child results in notions such as food that *tastes* good *is* good; and, if you like it, it is good for you. They believe their thoughts are the only thoughts possible and are, therefore, correct. Their cognitive structures are not merely less experienced and immature replicas of the adult's cognitive structures; the thinking processes of preoperational children are different in kind. They may be able to memorize large amounts of "nutrition" information, but their ability to understand the invisible and abstract nutrient and the changes it undergoes as it contributes to our health is beyond their reach. Moreover, their rapidly expanding verbal ability often enables them to recite facts and to use phrases that can lead adults to think that they comprehend more than their cognitive structures could possibly allow. For that reason, it is inappropriate to spend great amounts of time teaching facts about nutrients or food groups.

To illustrate the body's need for food, one teacher whom the authors observed told the children that their bodies were like machines and when they ran out of fuel (food), they would run down, stop, be unable to go again until they were refueled; if they were tired and run down, eating would restore their energy and make their feet fast. Imagery is an appropriate means of helping children conceptualize how food is used by their bodies. However, the teacher might have carried the lesson further by telling them that the machines ran most efficiently on "high test."

Adults working with prelogical children must occasionally rely on rote teaching techniques and conditioning to help children discriminate between foods that should be eaten regularly (high-nutrient density) and foods that should be eaten only now and then (low-nutrient density). It is always more beneficial to concentrate on foods that are healthful rather than to warn children of foods to avoid. A few beginning conditioning activities are given below. Many more exist in a variety of teacher resource books, some of which are listed in the Resource Lists at the end of this chapter.

Sorting. Provide children with pictures of familiar objects to sort into "food" and "not food" groups.

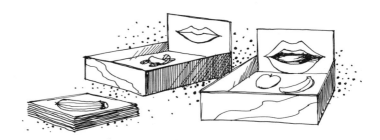

Junk food boycott. Involve parents in a junk food boycott for a week. Send home a list of foods that are low in nutrients to serve as a guide.

Nutrition workshop. Have a nutrition workshop for parents. Include some of the topics presented in Chapter 7.

Use puppets. Make a puppet from a large grocery bag with a see-through window at the stomach level. Feed it pictures of foods which are fad foods for a week. The following week, empty the puppet, and feed it nutritious food pictures. Parents can help to search for these pictures and send them in with their children.

Involve children in planning. Plan a menu to be served at lunch-time. Use a picture wheel of the four food groups made from a pizza board. Help children to choose the correct number of foods from each category to make a balanced meal.

Salt and sugar contents. Involve the children in the tracing tray activity described in the first section of this chapter under Food Properties. Encourage them to sort pictures of foods which taste sweet and foods which taste salty. Have them place foods, or food pictures in order, ranging from those that are a little sweet to those that are too sweet. Help them identify which foods are naturally sweet and which foods have had sugar added.

Good food makes things grow well. Plant beans in clear plastic cups with rocks or sand at the bottom for drainage. Put the beans against the plastic so that children can observe the emergence of the sprout and the progress of the roots. Feed one plant water only, one plant sugar water, and in one plant bury a small (1-inch square) of fish a few inches from the plant, preferably also against the plastic for easy observation. Observe the growth of all three plants. Discuss the color of their leaves, size, and rate of growth. Experiment with other plant foods. Avoid using standard plant fertilizers, however, since children already think that vitamins are pills or are added to foods.

BIOLOGIC ORIGINS OF FOODS

Some experiences that enable young children to develop concepts related to where and how foods originate are described in this section. In the next section, as we discuss helping children explore the ways in which foods are processed, they can begin to differentiate between foods that are highly processed and foods found or presented in their natural state.

Make a sprout farm. Allow each child to care for an individual baby food jar of alfalfa or mung sprouts for the period of one week. The sprouts must be started on Monday to be ready to eat at snacktime on Friday. See Figure 6-2 for directions. At snacktime, the sprouts can be eaten with or without dressing, mixed with a salad, or even served on a peanut butter sandwich! We observed one classroom that had an ongoing sprout farm; most of the children cultivated their own jar of sprouts every week. The seeds and measuring spoon were made available in the science corner of the room, and on Fridays the children who had sprouts either ate them with their regular snack or used them for barter!

Chart the growth of a bean. Place a lima bean, with a damp paper towel (folded) into a ziplock bag. Hang it from a line stretched across the window frame and watch it sprout. In a few days, mark the daily growth

FIGURE 6-2

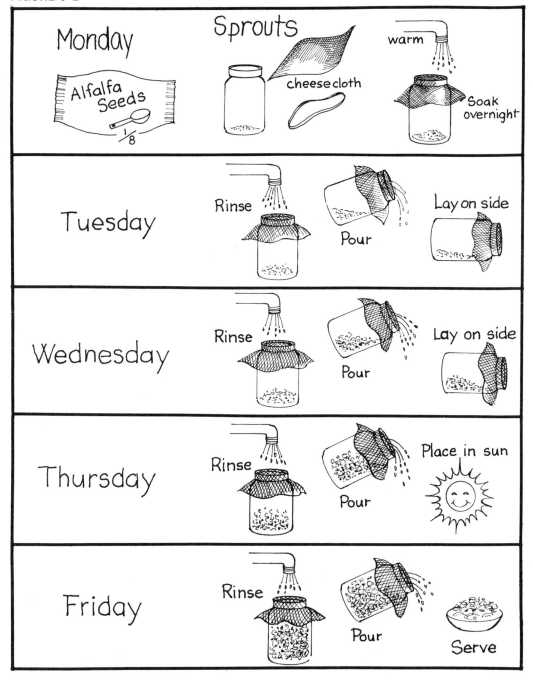

of the sprout with a black, permanent-ink magic marker. Add new lines to record the rapid growth every day. This activity is more interesting to the children if each child has a "bean baggie" to observe. Children can mark the growth on their own bags with this approach. Don't forget to serve bean soup as an extended activity (see the recipe for Jack's Soup in Chapter 5).

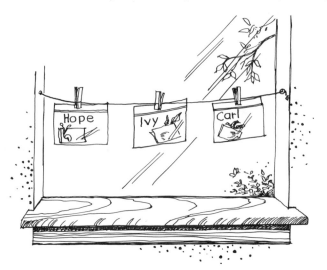

Explore peanuts. If possible, go to a peanut farm and with the permission of the farmer, pick up enough peanuts to roast, eat, plant, and make peanut butter for snacktime.

To make peanut butter, simply blend a cup of roasted peanuts with a little oil. If a food processor is used instead of a blender, it will not be necessary to add oil to the peanuts. Try mixing other ingredients with the peanut butter, like coconut, wheat germ, or sesame seeds.

Planting peanuts is a delightful project too. Be sure to send a few peanuts home with the children along with directions for planting them. Parents are often surprised to see how peanuts grow.

Make a peavine tent. Pound a large circle of 1-foot-long stakes into the ground. In the center of the circle, pound a tall pole (about 5 feet long). Attach strings to each stake and stretch them to the top of the center pole. Plant peas, beans, or climbing cucumbers at the base of each stake. As the vines grow, train them to wind along the string. This makes a cozy outdoor hide-out from which the children can observe vegetables growing on the vine. Variation: Pound about 6 stakes, 1 inch apart, in a straight row parallel to a fence (the row should be about 5 feet from the fence). Stretch the string from the stakes to the fence at an angle. The vines, when trained up the string, will make a lean-to tent.

Grow a windowsill garden. Sprout the tops of pineapples and carrots by setting them in damp sand in a jar lid; grow sweet potato vines by submerging one end of the potato in a jar of water. Stick toothpicks all

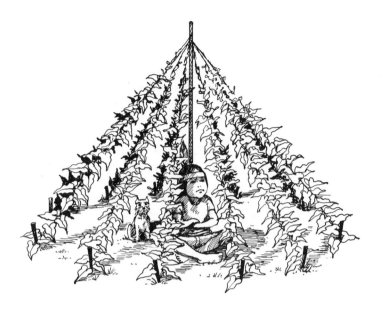

around the center of the potato and rest them on the rim of the jar to hold the top half of the potato out of the water. Another good potato project for a windowsill garden is to plant the "eyes" of Irish potatoes in cups. Later they can be transplanted in a garden or compost pile. When the vines die late in the summer, the potatoes can be harvested by the children. If the potatoes are sprouted at school, children can transplant their vines at home.

Visit a chicken farm. Buy some "family eggs" (fertile eggs) to incubate. After 21 days in the incubator, chicks will hatch from the eggs. While

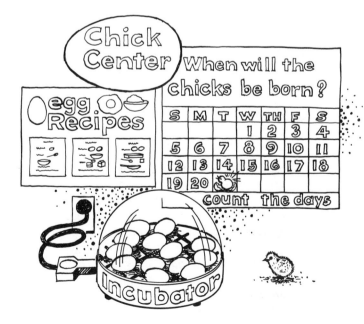

you are there, buy eggs to boil, poach, scramble, or fry at snacktime. Or use the recipe for Pickled Pink Eggs in Chapter 5.

Go fishing. Take the children with you. (Be sure to get some help from other adults with this project, however.) It may be necessary to supplement the catch with some fish from the market. Fillet and fry the fish in strips for a snacktime treat.

Have a clam roast. Furnish enough clams to allow each child to clean and steam one for a snack. The shells can be used for art projects.

Visit a dairy farm. Watch the cows being milked. Buy some cream to make butter and some milk to make cottage cheese. See the recipes for butter and Miss Muffet's Favorite Snack in Chapter 5.

Visit the farmers' market. Buy some fresh vegetables and fruits for snacktime. Whenever possible, visit a farm or orchard to "harvest" a snack for the group.

Visit a food cooperative. Have some wheat kernels ground while the children watch. Use the flour to make bread. Read *The Little Red Hen* for an extended activity. (See the Resource Lists at the end of the chapter.) It may be possible to borrow a grinder from the co-op to grind corn so the children can make corn bread.

Grow a garden. Label each row with a picture of the food that is growing in that row. On the picture, indicate whether the food will grow from a vine, from the root, from a stalk, or on a bushy plant. On a calendar draw a food picture to indicate the approximate date when each of the foods will begin to ripen for the harvest. Encourage children to count the days or months and to check the progress of their plants. If this activity is done in a center or school where children go home for the summer, have a get-together, perhaps a watermelon feast in the late summer and serve watermelons from the garden.

FOOD PREPARATION

Most often children's first encounter with a food is as a finished product presented on the table or on a shelf at the grocery store. Most preschool children think that vegetables "come from" the grocery store. They seldom have an opportunity to observe the processes that are involved in preparing food so that it can be stored on the shelf for long periods of time. Some of the processes involved in the preparation of food for storage are explored in this section. A trip to the grocery store to look at canned, frozen, and dried foods would provide a meaningful introduction to the activities that are presented here.

Freezing. Squeeze fresh citrus fruits to make juice. Freeze the juice in individual cups with sticks to make popsicles. Make other fresh fruit popsicles by mashing or squeezing the fruits and pouring them into ice trays or freezing them in paper cups. Yogurt can be added for variety.

Canning. Make jam or jelly. Read *Bread and Jam for Francis* by R. Hoben (See the Resource Lists at the end of the chapter.) Use the spread for snacktime in combination with whole-wheat bread or crackers, peanut butter, or homemade butter.

Dehydrating foods. Tape a carrot to a piece of cardboard. Trace around the carrot, and write the date on the cardboard. As the carrot shrinks, continue to measure and record dates. Stimulate the children to think about what is making the carrot shrink by asking questions like, Why is the carrot getting smaller? Where does the water go when it leaves the carrot? Refrain from "feeding" them answers, but instead, allow them time to wonder. Extend this activity by putting a small amount of water in a clear plastic cup on the windowsill. Mark the water level on the cup with a permanent-ink magic marker and record the date. Each day check to see if the water level has changed. Place new marks on the cup as the water evaporates.

Make a carrot necklace. Let the children wash the carrots, cut them into wheels, and string them to make a necklace or bracelet. Then hang them from the windowsill in direct sunlight until they are completely dried. They can be worn or cooked in a soup.

Make raisins. Materials: Fresh ripe, firm, seedless Thompson (or muscat) grapes; large bowl of water for washing grapes; paper towels on which to drain and pat them dry; a screen rack like those used for spatter painting; and a piece of cheesecloth, slightly larger than the rack, for a cover. Procedure: (1) Wash the grapes in the container of water. (2) Lift them gently from the water and blot them dry with towels. (3) Remove the grapes from the stem and spread one layer on the rack. (4) Cover the grapes with the cheesecloth and place them in direct sunlight to dry. The air must circulate over and under the tray for about four days. (5) Test the grapes by squeezing them. If they are dry enough, they will spring back when squeezed and leave no water on your fingers. They should be pliable and leathery. Eat them for snacks.

Dried apples. Let children wash, peel, and core apples. Slice them thinly and soak them for a few minutes in an ascorbic acid solution to prevent darkening; remove and blot dry. Now spread them on the rack and follow Steps 4 and 5 for making raisins.

145　　　　***Pickling foods.*** Use the recipe for Pickled Pink Eggs in Chapter 5.

Other Food Preparation Activities

Allow children to participate in as many food preparation activities as possible. They should have frequent opportunities to scrub, peel, scrape, grate, grind, dice, slice, whip, blend, and stir. Moreover, see-through pots and oven doors should be used if they are available to allow children to observe the effect of heat on ingredients. Providing maximum opportunities for child participation is important. Remember, when adults prepare most of the foods, first-hand opportunities for children to learn are decreased. Too frequently, food preparation activities consist of the adults preparing the food while the children watch.

Each step in the process of preparing food should be thought of as an opportunity for learning. Even scrubbing potatoes provides opportunities for children to learn the importance of cleaning foods before cooking them. For example, let them wash some dirty potatoes. Show the children the dirt in the bottom of the sink. Ask them if we had not washed the dirt from the potatoes before we cooked them for our snack, where would the dirt have gone? Would we have eaten it, perhaps? Let them wash and rinse the potatoes until the rinse water is clean.

Snack centers, like the one described in Chapter 4, provide additional opportunities for simple food preparation, and the recipes in Chapter 5 can be reviewed to find those that promote dicing, grating, kneading, or peeling skills.

REVIEW ACTIVITIES

1. Visit a preschool or child care center, and interview 3 three-year-olds, 3 four-year-olds, and 3 five-year-olds. Ask them the following questions:
   a. Name some foods that are good for you.
   b. Name some foods that are not good for you.
   c. Why do you eat food?
   d. How does food help you?
   e. Where do eggs come from?
   f. Where does butter come from?
   Were their answers typical or preoperational thinking? Now find out what kinds of food experiences they have had (making butter, visiting a dairy farm, cooking) by asking their teacher. Do you think their responses were influenced by their experiences or by their lack of them?
2. Select four activities from this chapter and present them to a small group of children. Record the children's responses. What words did they use to describe smells, textures, and tastes?
3. After participating with children in one of the activities from this chapter, let the children dictate an experience story on a chart describing the activity. Or, if more appropriate, make a display of the children's work.
4. Correlate one of the activities from this chapter with a cooking project from Chapter 5.

SUGGESTED READINGS

COPELAND, RICHARD, *How Young Children Learn Mathematics*. New York: MacMillan, Inc., 1979.

KAMII, C., *Number in Preschool and Kindergarten: Educational Implications of Piaget's Theory*. Washington, D.C.: National Association for the Education of Young Children, 1982.

PIAGET, J., *Judgment and Reasoning in the Child*. New York: Humanities Press, Inc., 1964.

RESOURCE LISTS

Books with a Food Interest

Books can be a useful tool for stimulating interest in a subject, in this case, nutrition. Below is a list of books with a food interest. Each should be reviewed by the adult and, if selected, coordinated with other activities. For example, *The Carrot Seed* by Ruth Krauss can motivate children to explore the origin and properties of carrots. Extended activities could include planting some carrot seeds, sprouting the tops of carrots, making carrot sticks or wheels to eat at snacktime, shrinking a carrot, and making carrot juice with a juicer.

ALIKI, *My Five Senses*. New York: Harper & Row Publishers, Inc., 1972.

_____, *The Story of Johnny Appleseed*. Englewood Cliffs, N.J.: Prentice-Hall, Inc., 1963.

BENSON, HAROLD, *Boy, the Baker, the Miller and More*. New York: Crown Books, 1975.

BERENSTEIN, JANICE and STANLEY, *Big Honey Hunt*. Beginner Books Series. New York: Random House, 1962.

BRUNA, DICK, *The Egg*. New York: Metheun, 1975.

BULLA, CLYDE, *A Tree Is a Plant*. New York: Thomas Y. Crowell, 1969.

BURNS, MARILYN, *Good for Me: All About Food in 32 Bites*. Boston: Little, Brown & Company, 1978.

CARLE, ERIC, *Pancakes, Pancakes*. New York: Alfred A. Knopf, Inc., 1970.

_____, *The Very Hungry Caterpillar*. New York: William Collins & World Publishing Co., Inc., 1961.

FENTON, CARROLL JANE, and HERMINE KITCHEN, *Fruits We Eat*. New York: John Day Co., 1961.

GALDONE, PAUL (Illus.), *Little Red Hen*. New York: Scholastic Book Service, 1975.

GIBSON, M.T., *What Is Your Favorite Smell?* New York: Grossett & Dunlap, Inc., 1964.

GREENWAY, KATE, *Apple Pie*. London: Frederick Warne Co., 1886.

HAWES, JUDY, *Watch Honeybees with Me*. New York: Thomas Y. Crowell, Company, Inc., 1964.

HOBEN, RUSSELL, *Bread and Jam for Francis*. New York: Harper & Row, Publishers, Inc., 1964.

KIRKUS, VIRGINIA, *First Book of Gardening*. New York: Franklin Watts, Inc., 1956.

KRAUSS, RUTH, *The Carrot Seed*. New York: Scholastic Book Service, 1971.

MCBURNEY-GREEN, M., *Everybody Has a House and Everybody Eats*. Reading, Mass.: Addison-Wesley Publishing Co., Inc., 1961.

MCCABE, TERRANCE W., and HARLEY W. MITCHELL, *Animals That Give People Milk*. Chicago, Ill.: National Dairy Council, 1970.

MIVERICK, ELSA HOMELUND, *Little Bear*. New York: Harper & Row Publishers, Inc., 1961.

O'NEILL, MARY, *Hailstones and Halibut Bones*. New York: Doubleday & Co., Inc., 1961.

PAUL, AILEEN, *Kids Gardening: First Indoor Outdoor Gardening Book for Children*. New York: Doubleday & Co., Inc., 1972.

SCHECTER, BEN, *Partouche Plants a Seed*. New York: Harper & Row, Publishing, Inc., 1966.

SCHEIB, IDA, *First Big Book of Food*. New York: Franklin Watts Inc., 1956.

SCHOAT, G. WARREN, *The Wonderful Egg*. New York: Charles Scribner's Sons, 1952.

SELSAM, MILLICENT, *The Carrot and Other Root Vegetables*. New York: William Morrow & Co., Inc., 1970.

_____, *Seeds and More Seeds*. New York: Harper & Row, Publishers, Inc., 1959.

SENDAK, MAURICE, *Chicken Soup with Rice*. New York: Harper & Row, Publishers, Inc., 1962.

SEUSS, DR., *Horton Hatches the Egg*. New York: Random House, Inc., 1940.

_____, *Scrambled Eggs Supper!* New York: Random House, Inc., 1953.

SHOWERS, PAUL, *Follow Your Nose*. New York: Thomas Y. Crowell Company, Inc., 1963.

STEVENSON, ROBERT LOUIS, *A Child's Garden of Verses*. New York: Charles Scribner's Sons, 1905.

STONE, A. HARRIS, and PETER PLASCENCIA, *Plants Are Like That*. Englewood Cliffs, N.J.: Prentice-Hall, Inc., 1968.

TOLSTOY, ALEXES, *Great Big Enormous Turnip*. New York: Franklin Watts., Inc., 1968.

TRESSELT, ALVAN, *Autumn Harvest*. New York: Lothrop, Lee & Shephard Co., 1951.

_____, *Wake Up Farm*. Lothrop, Lee & Shepard Co., 1955.

TUDOR, TASHA, *Pumpkin Moonshine*. New York: Henry Z. Walch, Inc., 1962.

WISE-BROWN, MARGARET, *Big Red Barn*. Reading, Mass.: Addison-Wesley Publishing Co., Inc., 1965.

YEZBACK, STEVEN, *Pumpkinseeds*. Indianapolis, Ind.: Bobbs-Merrill Co., Inc., 1969.

Creative Activities Resource Books

ADELL, JUDITH, *A Guide to Non-Sexist Children's Books*. Chicago: Academy Chicago Ltd., 1976.

CROFT, DOREEN J., *An Activities Handbook for Teachers of Young Children*. Boston: Houghton Mifflin Co., 1975.

ELIASON, C., and LOA JENKINS, *A Practical Guide to Early Childhood Curriculum*. St. Louis: C.V. Mosby Co., 1977.

FLEMMING, BONNIE, *Resources for Creative Teaching in Early Childhood Education*. New York: Harcourt Brace Jovanovich, Inc., 1972.

FORTE, IMOGENE, *Nooks, Crannies, and Corners: Learning Centers for Creative Classrooms*. Nashville, Tenn.: Incentive Publications, Inc., 1978.

WANAMAKER, NANCY, *More Than Graham Crackers: Nutrition Education and Food Preparation with Young Children*. Washington, D.C.: National Association for the Education of Young Children, 1979.

Free Food and Nutrition Materials

American Dental Association
Order Section CAT 77
211 E. Chicago Ave.
Chicago, Ill. 60611

American Dietetic Association
430 N. Michigan Ave.
Chicago, Ill. 60611

American Home Economics Association
2010 Massachusetts Ave., N.W.
Washington, D.C. 20036

County Extension Offices
Check local phone directory

Federal Extension Service, U.S. Department of Agriculture
14th St. and Independence Ave., S.W.
Washington, D.C. 20250

U.S. Department of Agriculture Food and Nutrition Service
14th St. and Independence Ave.
Washington, D.C. 20201

National Dairy Council
630 N. River Rd.
Rosemont, Ill. 60018

Superintendent of Documents
U.S. Government Printing Office
Washington, D.C. 20420

chapter seven

sharing the caring
with **PARENTS**

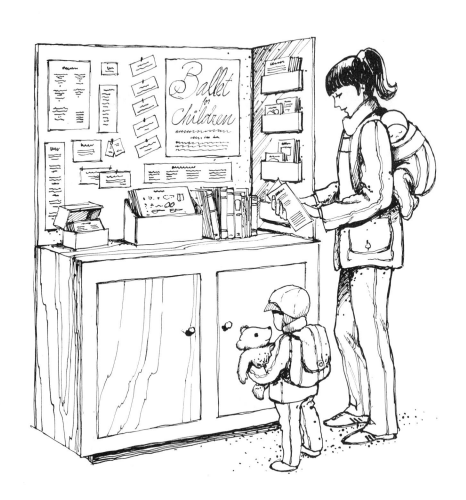

After reading this chapter the reader will be able to:

- Develop strategies for effectively communicating with parents regarding their child's nutritional needs.
- Plan a nutrition workshop for parents.

The traditional family in which the mother stays at home with the children and only the father works outside the home is now a picture from our country's historical past. In those days, children bounded down cold steps in the mornings, lured by the smell of bacon, eggs, and biscuits, to the prospect of a leisurely family breakfast. Mom or Grandmom fed the family, saw the children off to school and Dad off to work, cleared the dishes, and began to prepare the family's lunch. Most often, the children came home from school at lunch time if they lived close to the school or they ate home-packed lunches in sunny schoolyards. Since there were no school lunch programs, children's meals were prepared almost exclusively by their mothers. Obviously, keeping track of what children ate was easier when mother's job was mostly limited to the care and feeding of the family.

In contrast, one out of three babies born in the 1980s will have a mother who works away from the home during the baby's first three years of life. In 1983, more than half of the mothers of school age children worked, and that number is expected to increase. Many mothers now have career goals of their own, or they work outside the home because both parents' wages are needed to meet family expenses. Rising divorce rates, likewise, have had the effect of increasing the number of women who work away from their homes to support their households. These mothers, in contrast to the mothers of the recent past, have a difficult time keeping track of their children's food intake and influencing their food habits. The reasons are obvious.

Most children now participate in school or center lunch programs and eat other meals and snacks in a variety of settings, prepared and supervised by a number of different people. They may eat breakfast at home and lunch at school. After school they may fix their own snacks at home or be served a snack at a sitter's home or at a child care center. Likewise, they may eat supper at home, at a sitter's home, or at a fast-food restaurant on the way home. Their daily meals are too frequently uncoordinated—a patchwork of afterthoughts and hit-or-miss plans.

In spite of the many recent changes in the overall sociological picture, however, children's needs for a balanced, coordinated nutritional program have not changed. Keeping track of their food intake and helping them to develop positive dietary habits are as important today as ever. Obviously, however, to accomplish this requires systems that differ from past, traditional means, since parents now share the responsibility for the care and feeding of their family with many others.

CAREGIVING PARTNERSHIPS

Parents and all other caregivers must form a communication partnership, woven delicately with trust, cooperation, and mutual interest in the child to ensure that the fabric of childhood is securely patterned. Meeting children's nutrient and nuturance needs requires those who care for children to seek creative ways to communicate with one another.

In spite of the obvious need for communication, however, many centers, schools, and home care providers, surprisingly, have no mechanisms for regularly communicating with parents regarding the dietary habits and nutritional requirements of children. Since both caregivers and parents must coordinate their menus to provide an adequate nutrient balance for the child, this is a serious oversight and one that could have negative consequences.

In a study by Smiciklas-Wright et al. (1979), 16 percent of the mothers surveyed were totally unaware of what was served to their children during the day at the centers where their children attended. Many parents assumed that breakfast was regularly served at the center; most often it was not. Caregivers likewise were unaware (but could sometimes guess) which children ate breakfast at home and which did not.

These are obvious examples of information gaps that can be easily rectified by developing a two-way information-sharing system, one in which reporting responsibilities are shared by both caregiver and parent. Such a system can be viewed as a teeter-totter; parents on one end and the child's caregivers on the other. Both must work to maintain balance for the system to work. This type of system not only helps to keep both parties informed but allows parents to share in their child's daily experiences by learning about the events that shape and mold the health, lives, and personalities of their children. And caregivers, with adequate daily information from parents, can give more responsive care.

The Caregiver's End
of the "Teeter-Totter"

The caregiver has the advantage of observing several different children grow and develop simultaneously. Unlike parents, who observe their child more or less in isolation, the caregiver has a basis for making relatively unbiased assessments of individual growth progress. And because parents have both the right and the need to share in the progress of their children, the caregiver should systematically record the progress of each child and regularly report findings and concerns to parents. Not only should developmental events be recorded, such as reaching behavior, creeping, crawling, and walking, but, likewise, the child's elimination habits and dietary responses must be carefully monitored and reported.

Parents need to know of their child's dietary intake, so that a nutrient balance can be maintained. If the child is an infant, the parent and caregiver will have to communicate closely to monitor the baby's response to new foods as they are introduced into the diet.

Parents also need to be appraised of the health status of their child. For example, if their child has diarrhea or is constipated, the frequency and consistency of the stool should be reported. Headaches, earaches, loss of appetite, listlessness, frequent bruising, and sleeping difficulties could be symptoms of oncoming illness, allergies, or emotional stress. With the practice of regular, systematic reporting, growth deviations and eating or behavior patterns that can have negative consequences can often be identified early and a corrective procedure begun.

The following goals can be accomplished if caregivers develop a systematic plan for getting information to parents: (1) to inform parents of eating, elimination, or other health or behavioral problems exhibited by the child during the day; (2) to monitor cooperatively the child's growth and development; and (3) to impart important nutritional education information to families for the purpose of improving the nutritional status of their children. Some suggestions for communicating with parents follow.

THE PARENT SPACE

The entrance to a facility which provides care for young children and support for their families should be inviting. The atmosphere should communicate the message, I'm here to be helpful; let's work together. Brief, eye-catching nutritional information, children's workshop schedules, inoculation schedules, and other pertinent information can be presented at the entrance in ways that can accommodate a rushed, harried parent. In the Parent Space, include the following:

Two-way message minder. This is a form that can be attached to a clipboard perhaps and hung where the parent can leave a daily message for the caregiver. The caregiver can likewise inform the parent of the child's

TABLE 7-1 Message Minder (Infants)

PARENTS

Child's name _____ Medication _____

Any change in diet for today? _____

Before coming, baby _____ drank entire bottle,   _____ ½ bottle,   _____ no bottle,

   _____ ate a good breakfast,   _____ ate small amount,

   _____ ate no solid foods.

Baby slept _____ normally,   _____ seemed restless,   _____ woke earlier than usual.

Any accidents (cuts, bumps, bruises)? _____

Notes (for example, spitting up more than usual, and so forth) _____

CAREGIVERS

FOOD INTAKE			BOWEL MOVEMENTS		MEDICATION		NAPS
time	solids	liquid (oz.)	time	consistency	time	amount	time
A.M.							
P.M.							

Developmental milestones _____

Special program activities or events _____

Notes (needs, such as diapers, and so forth) _____

nutritional intake, response to new foods, health problems, elimination schedule, developmental milestones accomplished, and otherwise share concerns and joys with the parent on a regular basis. See Tables 7-1 and 7-2 for sample forms.

Bulletin board. Post the day's menu; information about community food resources; public health services; diet groups; supplementary food programs; and short, direct messages to help make parents aware of how they directly influence the eating habits of their children. The bulletin board also provides a central place for "idea exchanges" to be shared by parents. Lists of overnight sitters; schedules of weekend community programs for children, such as language and music classes, or art shows; and requests for recipes that make spinach appealing to children are all examples of the kind of information that can be shared here.

TABLE 7-2 Message Minder (Preschoolers)

PARENTS

Child's name _____ Medication _____

Dietary restrictions? _____

Breakfast this morning was _____

Bedtime last night _____ Slept (check one) _____ well _____ fitfully

Any accidents (burns, bruises, cuts)? _____

Other _____

CAREGIVERS

Special accomplishments _____

Special program events, upcoming or past _____

Nap today _____hours/minutes long, _____ restful, _____ restless

Appetite _____ good _____ finicky, _____ no appetite

Items needed: (forms, change of clothes, and so forth) _____

Notes_____

Recipe file. A recipe file can include recipes that have been prepared by the children. Include their favorite lunch and snack recipes, picture recipes, and recipes that are high in the vitamins and minerals most likely to be lacking in children's diets, that is, vitamins A and C, calcium, and iron. Provide a pencil and paper for parents' use when copying the recipes.

Recipe and coupon exchange. Parents who discover creative ways to entice children to eat vegetables or unpopular foods may want to share their recipes. Likewise, parents who collect coupons may wish to exchange them with each other. These exchange activities help to introduce parents to one another and to promote friendships within the child care community.

Lending library. Books related to parenting, nutrition, and child development can be checked out by parents. And parents who have read interesting books may want to share these with others. A lending library could be established with the aid of a parent volunteer.

Games for learning could also be checked out of the lending library by the parent and used to reinforce skills and to stimulate conversation and parent-child interaction. Likewise, a new game or activity could be placed on a table near the entrance for the child and parent to play together as a means of broadening the parent's understanding of the curriculum and how children learn through play.

Weekly or monthly menu cycles. These should be posted or, ideally, sent home with the children, so that the parent can plan their meals to ensure a nutrient balance for their children.

Bag lunch menu helps. Menu ideas for bag lunches are difficult to think of when parents must pack them day in and day out. New ideas are always appreciated. These could be posted or sent home in a newsletter.

Licensing requirements in most states dictate that hot lunches must be served in programs for young children. In the programs that are exempt from this requirement, however, parents must pack lunches for their children each day. Planning a nutritious, balanced menu for a bag lunch is a real challenge, especially if the parent tries to avoid prepackaged cakes, potato chips, and other typical bag lunch fare.

Some of the following ideas will be helpful:

1. Prevent soggy sandwiches by packing each item separately, either in baggies or in recycled margarine tubs. Include items for sandwich making and for eating separately. (Some foods are more appealing to children if they don't run together or mix.) Children love unpacking a meal that has been packed in this way. Opening each container is a little like going on a treasure hunt! Be sure to help the child learn to close containers tightly, however, so that if leftover juicy items are returned home, they will not dribble out en route.

2. Dip all the fruit or vegetables that are likely to discolor into citrus juice before packing, to prevent them from turning dark.

3. Be sure to include a napkin, perhaps one that has been decorated, or on which a love note has been written. The napkin can serve as a tablecloth upon which all the ingredients can be laid out and organized for serious sandwich construction.

4. Use whole-wheat, rye, or pita bread. If white bread is used, be sure it is enriched. Other breads include tortillas; bagels; corn muffins; and zucchini, nut, and pumpkin breads.

SAMPLE BAG LUNCH MENUS

tuna sandwich with salad dressing, chopped celery, and raisins
apple rings with peanut butter spread
milk

peanut butter and banana sandwich
carrot curls
chopped prunes
milk

SEND HOME DAILY OR WEEKLY
LOVE NOTES AND MONTHLY NEWSLETTERS

The need to use this technique is illustrated by this all too frequent exchange between parent and child after a long day of separation.

"What did you do today?"
"Nothing. Played."
"Did you have fun?"
"Umm-humm."
"Tell me what you did."
"Aw, Mom! Nothing."

What working parent hasn't been frustrated by a child's unwillingness to describe even a small part of the day! Ironically, that very day, the caregiver may have gone to great trouble and expense to take the children to the zoo, involve them in planting a garden, or they may have even had an opportunity to observe the hatching of baby chickens! Just the same, children, it seems, almost invariably respond to parental requests for information with "Nothing," or "Not much," no matter how exciting their day has been.

Ways need to be found to communicate to parents what the children do during their absence and to stimulate conversation and interaction between them. When this is done, parents are less likely to feel left out, for they get to share vicariously in their child's experiences. Moreover, they are comforted by knowing that their children are involved in interesting and challenging activities during the day.

Brief notes that can take many forms or newsletters are sure to be read and appreciated by parents and children. They can serve as a record of experiences shared with friends and can help stimulate conversation between adults and children. Likewise, they can be used to communicate important nutritional education information to parents.

Send newsletters regularly. In the newsletter, include recipes, nutrition activities to be completed by children and parents together, ideas for taking the drag out of bag lunches, sandwich ideas, snack recipes that can be made by the child, tips to improve the mealtime atmosphere in the home, ways to introduce new and different foods, and information on normal eating behavior for young children.

When sending newsletters, be sure to

1. Keep the information simple and interesting, but informative.
2. Include a section for parent input. They may like to share tips for packing good lunches or for interesting children in new foods.
3. Use appropriate seasonal or curriculum topics for the newsletter theme. Recipes, places to visit with children, finger plays, and simple activities should complement the chosen theme.
4. Send the newsletter home at the same time each month. Consistency heightens anticipation.

Send brief notes, for example, "Warm Fuzzies."[1] These could take the form of little slips of paper, either handwritten or mimeographed, which contain messages like, "I tasted an avocado today. We peeled it, cut it up, mashed it, and mixed it with mayonnaise and lemon juice. It was good on a Wheat Thin. When we go to the grocery store, we can look at some avocados together." Other messages might include ideas for introducing new or previously disliked foods, like combining them with dips or turning them into Popsicles.

GET-TOGETHERS AND INFORMAL ENCOUNTERS

Probably the best way to share information is face to face, a difficult task when parents work and their demanding and sometimes inflexible schedules leave little or no time to volunteer in centers or schools or even to attend conferences or workshops. There are ways, however, to maximize the number of encounters and improve their quality. These times spent together informally, as well as formally, are valuable and greatly beneficial to children.

During parent conferences, open house, afternoon pick-up times, or through a car window in the mornings, information can be shared that can improve the child's nutritional status if the caregiver is available and responsive. Parents conversing about lunchtime, for example, are often surprised and delighted to hear that their child has eaten tomatoes prepared in an especially appealing way. They may ask for the recipe. Caregivers, likewise, can glean important information effortlessly during informal encounters. The following dialogue between caregiver and parent reveals an example of how home meal pattern information was learned without the aid of a survey or more formal technique.

"Guess what happened to my youngest this morning, Mrs. Hillard?" the caregiver said laughingly. "She was helping to serve the cereal and used the dog's bowl instead of her own! Do similar things happen during breakfasttime at your house?"

"We rarely eat breakfast at our house. Shelley is usually too cranky to eat in the mornings anyway. All she will eat is Sugar Crunchys from the box on the way here. Got any ideas?" Mrs. Hillard replied.

Not only did the caregiver in this episode gain information from the parent that shed light on why Shellie is cantankerous most of the morning until snacktime, but he had an opportunity, at the parent's request, to share ideas for improving Shelley's overall dietary intake. Informal encounters like this can lead to productive and beneficial action. Some techniques for maximizing their number and quality are described below.

Be available at drop-off and pick-up times. Because some children stay in centers all day long, from early morning until evening, often longer

---

[1]Warm Fuzzies are "strokes" given to make people feel good. The term was first introduced in a program for social development called T.A. (Transactional Analysis) for Tots that was developed by Alvin M. Freed.

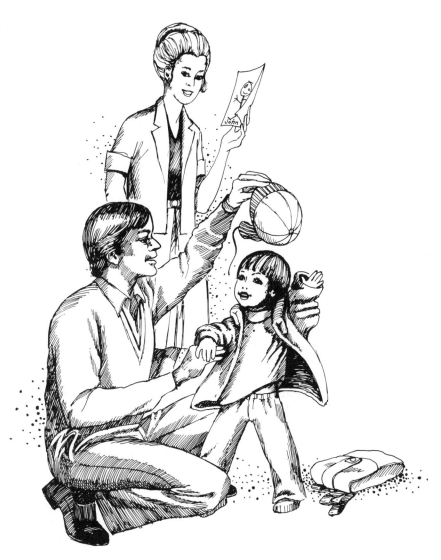

than the time spent there by some of their caregivers, it is often impossible for the "morning person" to inform the "afternoon" or "evening person" of significant events that should be reported to the parent at pick-up time. For this reason, significant events should be recorded by caregivers, perhaps on the message minder form before leaving, and they should be reviewed by the next caregiver before parents begin to arrive to pick up their children. With this practice, the caregiver can be prepared to discuss problems and demonstrate to the parent that continuity of care has been provided.

Few things are more anxiety provoking than to get home and discover an unreported bruise or laceration on a child. Likewise, if during the reading of a cozy bedtime story the child reports that he "threw up" at lunchtime, or had stomach cramps after eating a snack, the parent will resent not having been told. Therefore, parents should be required to come in when they pick up their children. Moreover, they should enter the facility with their children in the mornings to respond to the questions on the message minder before leaving. Caregivers should be prepared to spend a few informal moments with them, previewing scheduled events, reporting past occurrences, or just chatting if possible.

If the parents are not rushed in the morning or evening, they should be invited to watch or join in children's play.

Invite parents for lunch or snacktime. Give parents an open or at least occasional invitation to eat lunch or a snack with their children. What better way for parents to observe and learn what is normal eating behavior for young children! Moreover, caregivers can model positive ways for parents to interest their children in trying new and unfamiliar foods. Many times parents are amazed to see their children eating foods they would not consider eating at home.

Use the telephone. The telephone should be used to share something wonderful that the child has accomplished or occasionally to communicate a concern. This system is superior to sending notes when there is a problem to discuss. Notes allow for little or no feedback from the parent and therefore frequently promote frustration. Ideally, caregivers should try to contact the parents of their charges once a month to share positive information. What a nice surprise for parents who are too often conditioned to expect negative information about their child from telephoning caregivers and teachers!

Parent conferences. These may or may not be scheduled on a regular basis. They can be used to communicate developmental progress or to explore solutions to a problem that the child is experiencing. For example, potty training techniques can be standardized between the home and center to ensure success. Likewise, findings on a dietary recall or deviations in a child's growth patterns may indicate the need for a referral to a nutritionist or health care professional.

At each conference, the problem, if there is one, should be clearly defined, free of assumptions and judgments, and the parent and caregiver should work together to identify alternative solutions. Great care should be exercised to avoid confirming a parent's sense of inadequacy. Neither parents nor children are benefited when the caregiver or teacher assumes the role of the "expert" with all of the answers. Skilled and sensitive caregivers will seek ways to involve the parent in problem solving and to increase the parent's feelings of competence.

Begin a parent volunteer program. It is increasingly difficult to find parents who have the time to participate in a volunteer program on a regular basis. However, occasionally parents can come in to help with a particular project. Cooking, snack making, and some of the food-related projects described in Chapter 6 are ideal for parent participation. While taking part in them, the parents' interest in providing appropriate food experiences is often extended.

Have a nutrition workshop. Even though parents and caregivers may know about basic nutrients and how they influence health, and even though they may be able to verbalize the importance of choosing a variety of nutritious foods and know how to write a balanced meal plan, research reveals that this knowledge is not necessarily converted by them into sound dietary practice. An "application gap" has been found to exist between what is *known* about nutrition and what is *practiced* in homes and in facilities that feed young children. To illustrate, in a study by Smiciklas-Wright et al. (1979), parents and caregivers who were able to list nutritious snack foods when asked were found, in fact, to serve Kool-aid, candy, and pototoe chips to young children for snacks. Being able to identify nutritious snacks did not, in this case, guarantee that nutritious snacks would be served. Child care centers, however, were found to serve nutritious snacks more consistently than mothers at home, perhaps because of the necessity of long-range menu planning or the requirements placed upon those who participate in the U.S. Department of Agriculture food service programs.

Closing this application gap, then, should be the prime objective of any nutrition workshop. Nutrition education is one variable that has been found to be an effective means of altering nutrition attitudes and practices (Caliendo and Sanjur, 1978). Surprisingly, socioeconomic background and education levels appear to have little effect on the ability of a person to apply nutrition information.

Ways will have to be found to make it easier and more desirable to serve nutritious foods than to serve the usual high-calorie, low-nutrient fare. This is a tall order. To provide this information and motivation in a nutrition workshop is likewise a challenge.

Before beginning any nutrition workshop, it is wise to become acquainted with the dietary habits of the families who will attend. This can be done through the use of a survey or more or less informally over a period of time. The purpose of gathering this information is not so that you can work to try to get parents to change their diets, but just so that you will have a better understanding of the practices of the group for whom you are planning.

It is unwise to try, in a nutrition workshop, to change or alter drastically the dietary patterns of the families whose children are being served. Research shows that change in dietary habits come slowly, if at all, and the only recommended changes that are likely to be acceptable are those that do not differ radically from traditional diets. Therefore, the more subtle the suggested change, the more likely it is to find acceptance. For example, a switch from white flour to corn or whole-wheat flour for tortillas is a relatively small change or a switch from animal to vegetable fat for frying would be more acceptable than not serving fried foods altogether, particularly for the Mexican American family.

It is important to remember that there are many different types of diets that can and *do* adequately meet the nutritional needs of children and families, diets that are often unlike your diet. Frequently, the diets of children include food and food combinations that are unfamiliar but are nevertheless nutritionally sound. It is necessary to have an adventuresome spirit and an open mind and be ready, like the children, to explore and to be accepting of new cuisines.

Becoming familiar with the diets of families provides only a partial picture of a family's dietary practice. There are perhaps as many different ways of serving meals in the home as there are different diets represented. For example, not all children gather around the table with their families for meals. Frequently, meals are served by children from a single pot on the stove, left there by a working parent, or are prepared by an older child. Occasionally, there are not enough chairs or utensils for all family members to eat together or even enough pots and pans to cook more than one dish at a time.

Knowing the context in which meals are served enables the caregiver to present nutrition information with more sensitivity and to make suggestions that will be more useful for the families who attend.

No matter what a family's food preferences or practices, most parents will enjoy getting together during the evening hours with other parents who share common concerns, particularly if baby sitters are provided! Keep the workshop on a light, friendly note with much time for conversation and story sharing. Allow and provide opportunities for parents to get to know one another. This promotes a feeling of community and encourages sharing behavior and cooperation. As a bonus, provide a nutritious snack, preferably one that can be made while using a picture recipe. Talk about all the possibilities for learning that exist when food preparation activities are shared with children. Show parents how to make a snack center for their children to use independently at home; give them a list of inexpensive snacks that children can make or that children like, and introduce them to a variety of new recipe books for children. (See Suggested Readings at the end of Chapter 5.)

Other ideas include sharing practical suggestions on how to shop wisely on a limited income, guidance in how to obtain food stamps, and information on how one can participate in the WIC (Women, Infants, and Children's) program. Some additional topics for workshops include

- How to use label information for smart shopping
- Shopping with coupons and the art of refunding
- Taming the finicky eater
- How to select and prepare fresh foods
- Recipe sharing for those who cook for children on restricted diet
- How to make home-made infant foods
- Cooking to retain nutrients
- Overcoming a fear of vegetables and other "yuckey stuff"

It is known that parents frequently exclude certain items from children's diets because (1) the food has previously been rejected by the child, (2) the food is too expensive, or (3) the parent does not like or know how to prepare the food. Obviously, most of these reasons are areas that can be dealt with at a nutrition workshop. By considering them and the information gained by getting to know the food practices of the children you serve, you can plan a nutrition workshop that is mutually beneficial.

The three techniques that were discussed in this section—creating a parent space, sending home newsletters and brief notes, and arranging for parents and caregivers to get together formally and informally—all combine to reassure the parent that the physical needs and the emotional needs for acceptance, warmth, and affection of their children are being met. Moreover, they provide opportunities for caregivers to have an impact on the overall quality of children's health and well-being.

Caregivers, too, are in need of gaining information from parents that will enable them to provide truly responsive care. Parents bear an equal responsibility for maintaining a balance on the communication teeter-totter, and the information they can provide is of equal importance.

The Parent's End of the Teeter-Totter

Getting small children up, dressed, fed, and ready for a day away from home is no small feat, particularly if parents too are preparing for work. By the time the parent's car rolls up in front of the caregiving home, center, or school, the parent is most often caught up in a frenzied rush to be off. Requiring them at such a time to park the car, walk with their child into the facility, and take a minute to leave the necessary information on the message minder is difficult. However, without such a ritual, providing optimum care is impossible. It will be necessary to find ways to make it easy for them and to let them know how the information they provide helps to improve the quality of care for their children.

It is necessary to communicate daily with parents of well children, and obviously, communicating with the parents of children who are ill or who have special dietary restrictions or handicapping conditions will require additional communication efforts.

WELL CHILD INFORMATION

As mentioned previously, drop-off and pick-up times can be ideal for chatting and exchanging information. Occasionally, however, when parents arrive, the caregiver may be tending to or cleaning up after a sick child, or trying to contact its parent on the phone to determine whether or not the child was sick during the night. Obviously, chatting at such a time is out of the question. And realistically, there are many mornings when chatting with parents is impossible. This is why the message minder system is needed to provide continuity and regularity.

The message minder. This form was described previously in this chapter. It should be made easily accessible to the parent, perhaps by the doorway, and if the facility is large, each group's message minder should be color-coded for easy identification. With this system, both caregiver and parent can easily and quickly check off the requested information. If a new food is introduced into the infant's diet at home, the caregiver should be alerted in the comment section. If the parent wishes for the caregiver to introduce a new food to an infant, the food and the amount should be noted on the form. If a child failed to sleep well or if some catastrophic event occurred, like the death of a family pet or the hospitalization of a family member, the information should likewise be shared to aid the caregiver in coping appropriately with the child's possible "acting out."

It is particularly important to note whether or not the child ate breakfast before leaving home. Unfed children and children who have been fed nutritionally inferior foods may literally seem to run out of steam by mid-morning. They may become whiny or unable to participate in the morning's activities. The caregiver will need to have something nutritious on hand for these children. If the children regularly arrive in this state, it may be necessary to charge extra tuition so that breakfast can be regularly served to them. A request for breakfast information should be included on the message minder.

Food intake form. The information on this form (see Chapter 1, Table 1-6) can be filled out during a nutrition workshop or at the home of the child. If it is sent home, it should be sent early in the week to ensure a better rate of return.

With this information the menu planner can plan meals that reflect an awareness of and respect for the cultural preferences of the children who are served. This practice helps to build rapport with the parents. Furthermore, a complete picture of the family's nutrient intake enables you to plan meals that enrich the overall diets of the children.

Medical intake forms. These forms are required in most programs that care for young children. They alert the caregiver to possible health problems that affect children's diets, like allergies, metabolic disorders, diseases, and handicapping conditions. When this information is received, a list should be made detailing feeding instructions and listing the foods that children cannot eat. This list should be prominently displayed near the food preparation area and it should be updated frequently.

SPECIAL PROBLEMS REQUIRING AN INCREASED FREQUENCY OF COMMUNICATION

The ill child. The policy in most facilities which serve young children is to send children home when they become ill. As a result, already overtaxed parents lose income and frequently their jobs. To avoid this occurrence, desperate parents are often less than truthful about the condition of their child's health, a practice which, of course, results in delayed treatment and, consequently, a more severe illness. It is true that most facilities are not equipped to care for severely ill children, for severely ill children need continuous, quiet care. Children with some forms of mild illnesses, however, can occasionally be cared for without detriment to the other children, if a center is well-run and well-staffed. When children are not crowded in close, stuffy quarters, and caregivers are meticulous about sanitary procedures, practicing fastidious diapering and handwashing, isolation may not be necessary (Loda, 1978). When isolation is not a standard practice, parents are more apt to communicate concerning their child's illness.

Most illnesses require some dietary modifications, which should be practiced under the direction of the parents. Children with fevers need an increased caloric and fluid intake. Likewise, children with diarrhea need to discontinue milk and solid foods for a day or so and to increase their fluid intake. It is especially important to maintain close communication with the parent during these times, giving specific reports and requesting them. The message minder could be used for this exchange, or you may want to develop a special form.

Other special problems requiring dietary restrictions. Occasionally, children are born with metabolic errors that require dietary modifications. In these cases, a doctor or dietitian should prescribe the diet and then inform the caregiver of it.

Likewise, many children have allergic reactions to certain foods, and their parents may request that you provide substitute foods for them or that they be allowed to send their child's food. An updated list of food allergies and the children who have them should be kept handy and adhered to, since some allergic responses are severe enough to cause illness and even death.

The child with weight problems. Both underweight and overweight children have dietary problems which can be best dealt with when the caregiver and parents communicate. If physical causes for underweight have been ruled out by a physician, the caregiver will then need to find out the mother's and father's attitudes toward foods, the emotional climate during mealtimes, mealtime schedules, the child's activity level, and other emotional factors like sibling rivalry. Some parent behaviors which frequently contribute to *underweight* are

1. Worrying about intake and communicating that anxiety to infants and young children.
2. Coaxing, force feeding, bribing.
3. Getting caught up in a "power play." Children use eating behaviors to control their parents and therefore mealtimes become times to "battle."
4. Arguing at the table, tenseness between family members, airing of family problems, and general discord at mealtimes.
5. Unrealistic expectations regarding serving sizes resulting in practices like requiring children to clean their plates before leaving the table. A full plate is overwhelming, even nauseating to a child who is not very hungry.

6. Modeling finicky, picky behavior for children. For example, talking about which foods are not liked in front of children encourages them to try to think of foods they will not eat.

7. Talking about what a "picky eater" the child is, as the child listens. Children often feel the need to live up to their labels. Their self-concepts are partly formed from other's impressions and descriptions of them, and they will include these labels in their image of themselves.

Generally, there are two reasons for *overweight:* (1) The child consumes more energy than is expended through activity or (2) there is a physiological malfunction. Although a physician's guidance should be sought in both cases, the caregiver and parent can do much to prevent overweight and to help control it if the overweight is caused by an energy output and intake imbalance.

It has been suggested that individual activity patterns may be inborn. Children who are by nature less active but who are encouraged to eat a diet that is average for children their same age may be consuming more than they need to maintain an ideal weight. The problem is compounded when adults

1. Use food as rewards or withhold it as a punishment.
2. Bribe children with desserts.
3. Praise children for cleaning their plates.
4. Think that a plump child is a reflection of their "mothering abilities."
5. Make milk available in a propped bottle as the child drifts off to sleep.
6. Use food as a pacifier.
7. Give children more simple carbohydrates than they need.
8. Allow them to spend long hours in front of the TV set or in other sedentary activities.
9. Fail to involve them in rigorous activities, sports, or hobbies.
10. Set a bad example.
11. Keep fatty, high-calorie, low-nutrient foods on hand. The parents of overweight children need to avoid having these foods in the house.

All of these behaviors can be dealt with little by little, and often indirectly, in nutrition workshops and conferences and by using the techniques for putting nutrition education information into the hands of parents. In order to know what information should be shared with parents, it will first be necessary to find out which of the behaviors outlined above may be contributing to overweight or underweight in the child. Much of this information can be gained by sending a survey form home with the child. It may also be helpful to direct parents with specific nutrition education needs to appropriate information sources.

THE HANDICAPPED CHILD

Many centers actively recruit children with handicaps. Excluding them gives other children an unrealistic view of the world, and including them educates children to be sensitive and caring. Moreover, handicapped children benefit from being in the mainstream.

Many handicapped children are on restrictive diets. Their medication may interfere with their body's ability to absorb nutrients, or their disability may limit movement which often causes problems with overweightness. Communicating regularly with their parents is necessary to ensure an optimal nutrition environment for them.

The primary goal in feeding handicapped children, after their nutritional needs are met, is to encourage the development of self-feeding skills. Because their swallowing skills are often immature, and gagging and bitting reflexes tend to cease at a later age than for normal children, special feeding procedures have to be undertaken. Parents need to inform you of how to best accommodate their child during mealtime, and they need to be informed regularly of their child's progress in the development of self-care skills.

Furthermore, the parent can provide valuable information concerning the child's particular disability and make suggestions that can result in more successful feeding and nutrition education experiences. They may also supply you with special spoons, chairs, and feeding utensils.

You should ask the parents of these children to provide information to help you understand the world from the handicapped child's perspective, a necessary skill if you are to help the child to develop nutrition concepts. Obviously, it would not be useful to describe foods in terms of their colors to a blind child. Children with other sensory or motor impairments need to have the nutrition education objectives modified to meet their needs too. Parents should be encouraged to provide information that will make the communication of nutrition goals more meaningful to their children.

Urie Bronfenbrenner (1974) has studied the effects of parent involvement in programs which mainstream handicapped children and concluded that

1. Parent involvement is the key to successful mainstreaming.

2. The consistency of care between the home and school is greater in programs where parent involvement is strong. In programs where there is less parental involvement, inconsistent care occurred, and the children are more likely to be disoriented.

3. Children in programs where parent involvement is high are more likely to retain newly learned skills and behaviors when the program is discontinued than children in programs with little or no parental involvement.

4. When parents are encouraged to participate actively in programs for their children, their participatory attitude alleviated fears and anxieties that caregivers had about being able to provide for children with special needs. The unwillingness on the part of many caregivers to provide care for those children is reversed when the level of involvement is great.

CONCLUSION

Communication is a vital element when a child's nutrition program is shared by several people. Without an adequate two-way system of communication, mistrust and misunderstandings frequently occur. Parents may view caregivers with suspicion, guiltily fearing that their children have been abandoned to a system that does not satisfy their need for nurturing, or, conversely, that if the caregiver is "a hugger," he or she will replace the parent in the affections of the child.

Caregivers too have doubts about parent's motives and frequently interpret the questions asked by parents to be criticisms or evidence that parents consider them incapable of providing competent care. Parents who fail to ask questions, however, risk that the omission will be viewed as evidence of indifference toward their children.

Caregivers and parents feel very protective toward the children for whom they care. When they are required to give them up at the end or beginning of the day to the other party, it is quite natural to evaluate the quality of the care they suppose the child will receive in their absence. This requires comparing one's own skills and affections with those of the other person. Because of these strong feelings of attachment—feelings that are a natural and necessary part of caring for children—barriers are often erected between the parties who most need to communicate. But these barriers must be whittled down for the benefit of children, since nurturance does not flourish on battlefields.

Establishing a two-way system of communication in which the parents and caregivers share equal responsibility is an important part of a nutrition education program. It is necessary to find ways to promote trust and rapport if optimum care for children is to be provided.

REVIEW ACTIVITIES

1. Visit a child care center and ask for copies of forms that are used to encourage an exchange of information between caregivers and parents.
   a. Compare the information obtained from those forms to the information that parents and caregivers need to provide an optimal nutrition program.
2. Locate a child care center or school in which handicapped children are mainstreamed. Ask about the parent's responsibility for providing care or information that will improve the quality of care.
   a. Observe the child's behavior and self-care skills during meal or snack time.
   b. Describe the special facilities and/or paraphernalia needed to promote independence in these children.
3. Visit any school or center and talk to the person whose responsibility it is to plan the menu.

    a. Ask how many children have identifiable allergies or other conditions that require special diets.

    b. What special preparations must be made, and what is the parent's responsibility? How is this information obtained?

4. Interview a parent who used child care facilities and ask them to discuss with you the topic of how the center meets their needs.

    a. Then interview the director or child care giver and ask the same questions.

    b. Write a comparable paper.

5. Conduct the same activity described above with a parent who uses a family child care system. How are the communication needs of both systems being met?

chapter eight

problem solving
in nutrition **PROGRAMS**
for young children

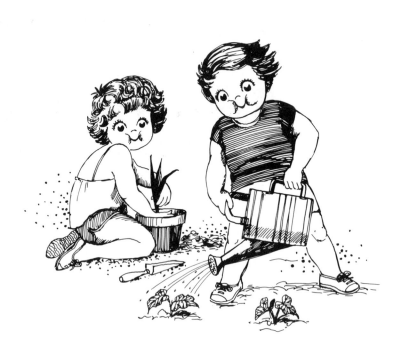

OBJECTIVES

After reading this chapter the reader will be able to:

- Solve nutrition problems that frequently occur in early childhood settings.
- Determine the accuracy of the nutrition information that is presented in mass media.

Today's consumer is regularly bombarded with so much nutrition information and misinformation that separating fact from fancy is becoming increasingly difficult. The fact is that exact relationships between some dietary practices and health are hard to establish, because of the obvious difficulties inherent in conducting research with human subjects.

Many dietary practices are known to be sound and basic, however. We have tried to present these in the earlier chapters of this book, combined with current theories of learning in early childhood and practical suggestions for implementation in programs. In this chapter, we discuss some common nutrition myths that impede the development of sound dietary practices. And we respond to some of the questions we are most frequently asked concerning appropriate nutrition strategies in programs for young children.

What can I as a caregiver do to help an obese child in my program?

You can provide the family with information on community resources and work with them to plan the best strategy for the child. Begin by suggesting that a doctor be consulted to determine if medical problems are a contributing factor. Then, if an examination reveals no medical problems, share the list of adult behaviors that can contribute to obesity in children given in Chapter 7. Research reveals that children from families with one or more obese parent have a 40 percent chance of becoming obese later in life and a 70 percent chance if both parents are obese (Moosberg, 1948). Although it is not known to what extent genetics influence obesity in children, we do know that certain adult behaviors can promote it.

While the child is in your care you can help by (1) studying the activity patterns of the child. Does he or she choose sedentary activities rather than gross motor activities? If this is the case, encourage more running, jumping, and climbing. (2) Study the eating behavior of the child. Is the child eating from the plates of other children, hoarding food, or "wolfing" it down? He or she may need to be distracted with lunchtime "chores." Slowing the rate of eating can reduce food intake. (3) Serve foods that are nutrient dense, low in calories, but high in other nutrients. (4) Keep in mind that the goal is not to help the child reduce, but to keep the child from gaining additional weight. As the child grows in height and if the weight is held steady, the child will grow within ideal range (see Table 1-3 for normal height and weight ranges). (5) Refrain from nagging or calling attention to the child's size in an effort to motivate the child to "see himself or herself as he or she appears to others." (6) Help to increase the child's self-esteem and feelings of worth and security by providing emotional support and warmth and by increasing opportunities for success and acceptance.

Should we serve foods with chemicals in them to children?

Would this food label listing cause you to shudder? *Ingredients:* water, starches, cellulose, pectin fructose, sucrose, glucose, malic acid, citric acid, succinic acid, anisyl propionate, amyl acetate, and ascorbic acid. These are some of the chemicals that make up a 100 percent natural, vine-grown cantaloupe. Potatoes contain about 150 different chemicals (at least one of them is poisonous to man when consumed in large quantities). Even mother nature's own milk consists of about 95 chemicals. In fact, all foods are chemicals; the people who eat them are composed of chemicals too.

Chemicals that are extracted from foods and added to other foods are called additives. Examples include sugar, salt, lecithin from soybeans, and gelatin from bones.

Sometimes chemicals are synthetic; they are produced in a test tube and added to foods. Surprisingly, our bodies cannot discriminate between those which are synthetic and those which are extracted from food sources. Our bodies are equally grateful or irritated by them.

Two popular natural additives—salt and sugar—account for 93 percent of all the additives we use in our food supply. They, like other flavorings, colorings, stabilizers, and purifiers, make it possible for the food industry to make a wide selection of food available to us year round at fairly reasonable prices. Unfortunately, additives also make it possible for the food industry to "invent" foods and then create a demand for them through the advertising media. Often these foods are nutritionally deficient imitations of foods and are used to replace the more nutritious foods that growing children need. The fact that identifiable nutrients such as vitamin C have been added does not make them the nutritional equivalent of the foods they mimic. In this sense chemicals that are used for additives can be harmful for you.

Even the term *natural* can be misleading. It is possible to create a completely new food by combining "natural chemicals" extracted from other foods. Therefore, a good rule of thumb is this: The further a food is from its natural-grown form, the less nutritious it is likely to be.

Shouldn't we substitute honey for sugar in children's foods?

Honey cannot be considered significantly more nutritious than granular sugar; the small amount of vitamins and minerals it contains is negligible. Moreover, measure for measure, honey has more calories than sugar: 1 tablespoon = 48 kilocalories; 1 tablespoon honey = 64 kilocalories. Its sticky consistency also promotes dental caries when the honey is not brushed away.

Back in the "olden days" when children had a sweet tooth, their parents supplied them with apples or other fresh or dried fruits. As their craving for sweets was satiated, they were simultaneously provided with the fiber and nutrients their growing bodies needed. Today, however, high-calories, low-nutrient sweets like candies, cakes, and cookies are too often given to children in place of other foods that they need for growth.

There are over 100 substances called *sugars*. They may be called *molasses, dextrins, glucose, sucrose, fructose, maltose, corn syrup lactose,* or *honey*, but sugar by any name is treated the same by the body. All are carbohydrates and when consumed in disproportionate amounts—that is, when the energy they provide exceeds the energy expended by the body—they contribute to obesity.

Should I add salt to the foods I prepare for children?

Probably not. It appears that a "taste" for salt is not predetermined but is, instead, acquired. Children are conditioned by the adults who care for them to expect a certain level of salt in their foods. Since four- to seven-month-old infants accept equivalent amounts of salted or unsalted foods when given a choice, we know that children can be conditioned early to expect foods to be just so salty; any more will be "too salty."

Taste is not always an adequate indicator of the level of salt in food, however. Surprisingly, one serving of cottage cheese contains as much sodium as about thirty-two potato chips! Even vegetables right out of the garden, meats, and water are natural sources of sodium. Meeting the body's sodium requirements under normal conditions is not difficult, given these salty sources. And since we know that sodium can contribute to hypertension in people who are genetically predisposed, it is a good idea to learn to season foods without using the saltbox. Consult Table 8-1 for ideas.

If you would like to know more about the salt content of foods, write for the publication, *Sodium Content of Foods,* from the Office of Governmental and Public Affairs, Room 507A, USDA, Washington, D.C. 20250.

TABLE 8-1   How to Season Food without Salt

	MEAT, FISH, AND POULTRY
BEEF	Bay leaf, dry mustard powder, green pepper, marjoram, fresh mushrooms, nutmeg, onion, pepper, sage, thyme.
CHICKEN	Green pepper, lemon juice, marjoram, fresh mushrooms, paprika, parsley, poultry seasoning, sage, thyme.
FISH	Bay leaf, curry powder, dry mustard powder, green pepper, lemon juice, marjoram, fresh mushrooms, paprika.
LAMB	Curry powder, garlic, mint, mint jelly, pineapple, rosemary.
PORK	Apple, applesauce, garlic, onion, sage.
VEAL	Apricot, bay leaf, curry powder, ginger, marjoram, oregano.
	VEGETABLES
ASPARAGUS	Garlic, lemon juice, onion, vinegar.
CORN	Green pepper, pimento, fresh tomato.
CUCUMBERS	Chives, dill, garlic, vinegar.
GREEN BEANS	Dill, lemon juice, marjoram, nutmeg, pimento.
GREENS	Onion, pepper, vinegar.
PEAS	Green pepper, mint, fresh mushrooms, onion, parsley.
POTATOES	Green pepper, mace, onion, paprika, parsley.
RICE	Chives, green pepper, onion, pimento, saffron.
SQUASH	Brown sugar, cinnamon, ginger, mace, nutmeg, onion.
TOMATOES	Basil, marjoram, onion, oregano.
	SOUPS
BEAN	Pinch of dry mustard powder.
MILK CHOWDERS	Peppercorns.
PEA	Bay leaf and parsley.
VEGETABLE	Vinegar, dash of sugar.

Reproduced with permission. © American Heart Association.

Is there truth in the old axiom, "Feed a cold, starve a fever"?

It is not a good idea to starve either a fever or a cold. When a child has a fever, the basal metabolic rate increases in portion to the rise in the fever, which, in turn, results in a demand for more calories. If the child can tolerate fluids other than water, it should be given liquids that contain sugar. Fruit juices, carbonated beverages, ice cream, and sherbet can provide the liquids needed by a child with a fever. Skimmed milk or, if it can be tolerated, whole milk and soups can likewise help to meet the body's extra demand for protein that is created by a fever.

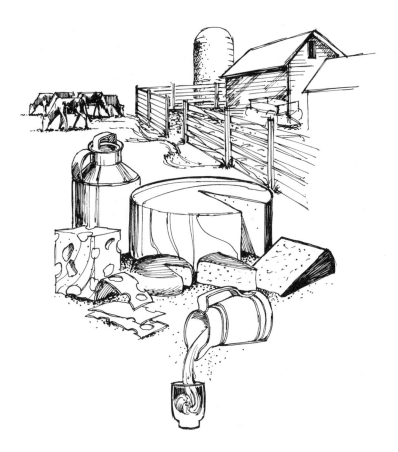

How much milk is enough?

Helping children learn to feed themselves is a messy, trying venture. It takes time, patience, and a sense of humor. For this reason, prolonging the use of the bottle for feeding is tempting. When milk is given in the place of meats, fruits, and vegetables, however, the child is deprived of important nutrients needed for growth—iron, ascorbic acid, and niacin, for example. When milk is consumed at the expense of other foods, intake should be curtailed. The child should be allowed no more than 24 ounces a day, unless all other foods are readily eaten and the child is not overweight. The toddler's RDA for calcium can be met by consuming 8 ounces of milk with additional servings of dairy products and frequent servings of green vegetables and legumes.

What should I do when infants and toddlers demand to be fed everytime they see me feed another child, even though they have just been fed?

"Monkey see, monkey do!" Nothing could more aptly describe how infants and toddlers learn. When one toddler sees another eating, he or she is stimulated to eat also, and hunger has little to do with it! It is best to distract the children who have already been fed with another activity. Obviously, in a group setting, infants cannot be fed every time they are stimulated by seeing another infant feeding. If possible, feed infants in a quiet place out of the visual range of other infants. This can be accomplished sometimes by the use of a small screen.

What is the best way to teach toddlers and young children mealtime manners?

1. Provide a good example.

2. Ignore inappropriate behavior as much as possible while reinforcing or otherwise giving attention to those behaviors that are more appropriate.

3. Have reasonable expectations. Children under the age of two, for example, who are learning to aim the spoon to their mouths without tipping it cannot be expected to remember to swallow before talking, chew with their mouths closed, or refrain from interrupting adult conversation. Likewise, infants can be expected to explore their foods with their fingers and to spit it out unceremoniously if it seems disagreeable to them.

4. Work on teaching only one new skill at a time, rather than picking and nagging at every infraction. If it has been determined that the child is mature and skilled enough to be successful, introduce a new skill or expectation and reinforce every effort to achieve it by smiling, nodding, or offering words of encouragement.

5. Be patient. Manners take time to develop. They must grow with the child and be nourished by a supportive, accepting environment.

Many of the children in my program eat at fast-food restaurants on the way home several times a week. Is that a good nutritional practice?

That depends on what they choose to eat and how frequently they eat it. Health professionals have traditionally criticized the levels of fats, sugars, and over-all caloric content of fast-food fare. Apparently, however, the nutrient levels of foods served in fast-food restaurants differ greatly. According to *Consumer Reports* (1979), Burger King's "Whopper" and McDonald's "Big Mac" are not nutritional equivalents; the amount of calories, fat, carbohydrates, sugars, sodium, protein, and other essential nutrients vary. Likewise, the nutrient content of meals served in popular chicken restaurants vary, and pizzas from some parlors are more nutritious than from others. Therefore, shopping for fast foods, like comparative shopping for other consumer items, requires a discriminating eye.

Average meals in most fast-food restaurants provide more than half of the RDA of calories required for most normal children and adults. Sodium levels are, at this writing, also high. An average meal provides more than half of the recommended amount of sodium needed by most people during a twenty-four-hour period and less than one-third of the RDA of other nutrients.

It has been estimated that the average American eats fast foods at least nine or ten times a month. This represents a substantial percentage of the young child's evening meals. Parents, tired after a day's work, stopping with their children on the way home from the center or school, may be easily worn down by children's demands for some of the less nutritious foods on the menu. Although forethought is difficult at times like these, meals should more or less be planned before arrival at the restaurant. In a nutrition workshop for parents, you might suggest this technique for improving nutrient food intake on those days: Suggest that children be presented with a choice of a few entrees (selected by the parent) from which the children will choose. If the menu is planned before arrival at the restaurant, the children will know what to expect. This eliminates the temptation to throw tantrums for shakes and sweets, which should be provided only rarely. When parents give in to tantrums, thrown most often when children sense that embarrassed parents are less likely to remain firm in a public place, children become tyrants. Their diets are then controlled entirely by them. Although it is important for children to have the opportunity to make choices, the foods from which they are allowed to choose should be controlled by adults. That can be best accomplished if it is done in advance.

I take care of a child whose family is vegetarian. If the child eats only vegetables and fruits in my program, will she be well nourished?

It is not likely, unless care it taken to combine the vegetables with legumes, nuts, and cereal grains to meet the protein needs of the child. Unfortunately, however, the proteins from these sources are not utilized by young children as well as they are by adults. Furthermore, vitamin B_{12} is found only in animal foods, and the deficiency takes from two and three years to develop, so the results of its exclusion are not readily apparent. If the diet merely excludes meat but not eggs, milk, or dairy products, meeting the nutritional needs of the child is less difficult. In any case, children on vegetarian diets need to have a special meal plan that can best be developed by consulting a nutritionist, and/or conferring with the parent. Vegetables and fruits alone do not contain all of the amino acids that are required for proteins to be utilized by the body. Therefore, a meal that has been planned for a group on a regular diet, but from which the meats and dairy products have been excluded for the vegetarian child, will not be adequate.

Is white bread as nutritious as whole-wheat bread?

If white bread has been made from enriched flour, that is, flour to which the vitamins thiamine, riboflavin, niacin, and iron have been added to replace those removed during the milling process, white bread is an adequate substitute. The trace mineral content in white bread is not as great as in

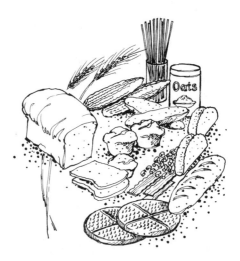

whole-grain foods, however. A few other nutrient differences exist also. The protein content of white, enriched breads is 8.7 grams, compared with the protein content of whole-wheat, which has 10.5 grams, for example. Moreover, whole-wheat bread generally has a little more iron and provides more fiber than enriched white breads.

What do I feed a child with diarrhea?

Diarrhea in an infant can be very serious, even dangerous, since it can cause a fatal dehydration. It requires the immediate attention of a physician. Dietary management requires that all foods be withheld, including milk. The child will need approximately 120 milliliters of liquid per kilogram of body weight a day. Therefore, water or weak tea should be given frequently. A carrot soup, prepared by diluting pureed (baby food) carrots with an equal amount of water (Foman 1974), can be introduced in the early stages, then later, as the condition improves, diluted skim milk (half strength), toast, gelatin, and cooked cereals can be gradually reintroduced, one at a time. When the diarrhea has ceased, whole milk or formula may be reintroduced, then gradually the other foods. If the condition recurs when solid foods are given, they should be withdrawn, and the procedure described above should be repeated.

Diarrhea can be caused by an allergy or a virus. In a center, it should be treated as though it is a virus unless a physician diagnoses it to be an allergy. That means fastidious diapering must be practiced for all children, not just with the ill child. Hand washing, yours and baby's, between every change, disinfecting the diapering table between every change, putting the soiled diaper in a closed container immediately (not first walking across the room with it) are a few basic diapering techniques that must be practiced when a diarrhea outbreak occurs.

Most state regulations require that children with diarrhea be isolated. Unfortunately, that practice sometimes causes center staff to relax diapering standards. Often the viral culprit is in the diaper of a child whose stool appears to be perfectly normal and is therefore treated with less caution.

What should I give a child who has just vomited? They usually beg for water or juice. Should I give it to them?

Probably not for at least two hours. This gives their stomachs a chance to "settle." After a few hours, if they can tolerate a little water, they may be offered some lightly flavored beverage like ginger ale. Later, they may want to try some toast or a cracker. Milk and other foods with a high fat content are not recommended until the child has been able to tolerate crackers, beverages, and perhaps skim milk.

I care for a child who will not eat at the center. What should I do to entice him to eat?

The first thing to do is to send a food intake form home with him (see Table 1–8). When it is returned, compare the menu he is used to with the foods that you have been offering him. Determine some things that could be prepared that might appeal to him, but don't make a fuss over it. If the child is well, he will eat when he feels comfortable enough in the surroundings, especially if the food seems somewhat familiar to him. If the child appears to be losing weight, however, he may not be eating at home either, in which case a conference with his parents is indicated. He may be ill or involved in an emotional setting at home that promotes poor dietary habits (see the discussion in Chapter 7 concerning underweight children). In any event, do not let his "not eating" behavior become an attention-getter or a means of manipulating you. Ignore it, but continue to think of ways to draw him into the mealtime experience. Preparing food with children, as described in Chapters 4, 5, and 6 is an excellent way of helping children get used to eating away from home and to learn to eat new foods.

I care for a child who eats dirt. He licks shoes, the floor, and literally eats it when we go outside. How do I deal with this?

Craving for pica is not uncommon in children with a nutrient deficiency. The child will need a dietary and physical evaluation. A referral to a physician is recommended.

I care for a child whose parents send the same foods day after day in their child's lunchbox. I'm concerned that the diet is not a balanced one.

The food prejudices of adults often influence what they serve to their children. If parents have a limited range of likes, their children will more than likely have been exposed to few foods. Unfortunately, this often results in an unbalanced diet, which can impact negatively on the growing child. Consult Chapter 7 for ideas for putting nutrition information into the hands of the parents. While the child is with you, use techniques described in Chapters 3, 4, 5, and 6 to introduce the child to new foods and overcome prejudices. Send recipes home with the child. Often, parents don't prepare foods because they are unfamiliar with them, or because they do not know how to prepare them.

Some of the children in my program bring snacks such as carbonated beverages, candy, cookies, and other foods that I consider nutritionally inferior for use at snacktime. How can I encourage the parent to send in more nutritious snacks? Some parents even send fruit punches in their infants' bottles!

Some people think that fruit drinks are nutritional equivalents for fruit juices. Unfortunately, most of these beverages are nutritionally equivalent to candies instead. The commercial advertisements for many of these products can be misleading to those who are not observant. Moreover, there is a direct relationship between the viewing of television advertisements and children's requests for the foods that have been advertised. A survey of children's weekend television programs in Boston revealed that a fourth of the food advertisements were for candy and related foods, a fourth were for cereals (mostly sweetened cereals), about 20 percent for fad foods and snack foods, and the rest for other foods.[1] Tired parents shopping with their children on the way home from the center or school are quickly worn down by children's persistent requests in the supermarket.

Therefore, it may be helpful to use some of the means described in Chapter 7 for communicating with parents to improve the nutritional status of their children. A steady stream of nutrition information sent home in short, interesting forms will be most effective. You might also involve them in a junk food boycott, or send a list of suggested nutritious snack foods home with the child, like the ideas for sandwich making given in Chapter 7. Often it helps to inform parents that nutrition is an important part of the curriculum in your program and that one program goal is to help children learn which foods are appropriate for lunch and snacks and which foods are not. Provide parents with a list of foods they can use to help you teach their child about nutrition. Encourage them to condition children to choose nutritious foods by providing them with these and using the others only occasionally.

To what extent are the food preferences and requests of children influenced by what they see on television?

They are influenced quite a lot. Research shows that young children cannot discriminate between commercials and regular shows. They all sort of blend together. One of the important developmental tasks of a preschooler is to learn to discriminate between fantasy and reality. This is a difficult task for them, and their problems are compounded by a tendency to literally

[1] F. E. Barcus, "Weekend Commercial Children's Television—1975" (Newtonville, Mass.: Action for Children's Televison, 1975).

interpret what they see and hear. Moreover, they do not identify subliminal intonation. A "fruit-like" drink is a fruit drink, for example (even adults have trouble here). People who are shown on television surrounded with friends, who have power or energy, or who are able to accomplish incredible feats after eating appealing foods shown larger than life, serve as models.

It has been proven that a direct correlation exists between the number of television commercials viewed by children and the frequency of requests they make for an advertised product. Therefore, it is desirable to view commercials with children, to aid them in becoming more discriminating viewers. Ask questions like, "Why is this mother giving her children this drink? Is it good for them? How do we know? Can we find out?" Typical prelogical responses will include, "Because they like it," "She wants her boy to have friends at his house; the friends will come if you give it to them, and it's good for them, if they like it."

Involve parents and children in a TV advertisement-viewing project. Ask them each to view several food commercials with their children and write down the main points the commercial seemed to be making. For example, did the commercial promise friendship, love, financial success, or power as a result of eating this product? What were the subliminal strategies used to rivet your attention to the product? Can the product deliver all that it promises?

Because the nutritional status of children affects their physical and mental growth, how can I determine whether or not children are developing on schedule?

A variety of factors can influence the young child's developmental schedule, either to accelerate or decelerate it. Nutritional status, sex, race, genetic factors, the condition and age of the mother during pregnancy, birth weight, environmental stimulation, and emotional security are but a few.

The norms given in Table 8-2 are fair indicators of optimal growth and development and can serve as a guideline for calculating individual development progress. (Height and weight charts are given in Table 1-3.) However, because the rate of growth and development differs considerably in small children, it is unwise to expect all children to reach the same level at a specific age. Tables and charts can be useful tools, however, for alerting the adult to possible problems or areas of concern. Developmental milestones accomplished should be recorded and shared with parents. Documented information can be used as a diagnostic tool for discovering developmental lags, which can sometimes be remedied with the aid of therapy or an improved diet.

For this reason, it will be necessary for the caregiver to cooperate with the parents in an effort to record developmental milestones as they are accomplished by the child. The first time an infant rolls over, pushes to his or her knees, or drinks from a cup should be recorded and the event shared with the parent. These records could help prevent future developmental problems, in addition to providing parents with a source of pleasure and pride in the accomplishments of their children.

TABLE 8-2 Landmarks of Development

PHYSICAL, MOTOR, AND LANGUAGE DEVELOPMENT	SOCIAL DEVELOPMENT
0–1 month	
Birth size: 7–8 pounds, 20 inches	Helpless
Feedings: 5–7 per day	Asocial
Sensory capacities: makes basic distinctions in vision, hearing, smelling, tasting, touch, temperature, and perception of pain	Generalized tension
Reflexes: sucks, swallows, cries, hic-coughs, grasps	
2–3 months	
Sensory capacities: color perception, visual exploration, oral exploration	Visually fixates on a face
Sounds: cries, coos, grunts	Smiles at a face
Motor ability: controls eye muscles, lifts head when on stomach	May be soothed by rocking
4–6 months	
Sensory capacities: localizes sounds	Expects feeding, dressing, bathing
Sounds: babbling, makes most vowels and about half of the consonants	Recognizes mother
Feedings: 3–5 per day	Distinguishes between familiar persons and strangers
Motor ability: controls head and arm movements, grasps, rolls over	No longer smiles indiscriminately
	Enjoys being cuddled
7–9 months	
Motor ability: controls trunk and hands, sits without support, crawls (abdomen touching floor)	Develops specific emotional attachment to one or more caregivers
	Protests separation from mother or chief caregiver
	Enjoys "peek-a-boo"
10–12 months	
Motor ability: controls legs and feet, stands, creeps, uses pincer grasp of thumb and forefinger	Expresses anger and affection
Language: says one or two words, imitates sounds, responds to simple commands	Expresses fear of strangers
Feedings: 3 meals, 2 snacks	Develops curiosity, explores
Size at one year: 20 pounds, 29 inches	Responds to own name
	Understands "no-no"
	Waves "bye-bye"
	Plays "pat-a-cake"

TABLE 8-2 Landmarks of Development

PHYSICAL, MOTOR, AND LANGUAGE DEVELOPMENT	SOCIAL DEVELOPMENT
1–1½ years Walks (10–20 months) Sits on chair with fair aim Builds 2–3 cube tower Makes lines on paper with crayon Has definite repertoire of words—more than 3 and less than 50 Progresses rapidly with understanding vocabulary	May be upset when separated from mother Obeys limited commands Makes no attempt at communicating information Shows no frustration at not being understood
1½–2 years Runs, kicks a ball May be capable of bowel and bladder control Has vocabulary of more than 200 words *Size at 2 years:* 23–30 pounds, 32–35 inches	Temper tantrums (1–3 years) Frequently does opposite of what is told Displays increased interest in communicating with others
2–2½ years Jumps into air with both feet Takes a few steps on tiptoe Can move fingers independently Uses 2- to 5-word sentences	Shows frustration if not understood by adults Imitates parents' actions Displays interest in other children Engages in brief periods of parallel play
2½–3 years Runs smoothly Uses short sentences *Size at 3 years:* 32–33 pounds, 37–38 inches	Grows possessive about toys Enjoys playing alongside another child Gives orders Insists on rigid sameness of routine
3–4 years Stands on one leg, draws a circle and a cross (4 years) Complete sentences of 6–8 words (4 years) Has become self-sufficient in many routines of home life *Size at 4 years:* 38–40 pounds, 40–41 inches	Displays intense curiosity, asks questions Plays cooperatively with other children Shows interest in other children's bodies (3–5 years)
4–6 years Skips, broad jumps, dresses self Copies a square and a triangle (5 years) Talks clearly, has mastered basic grammar, relates a story *Size at 5 years:* 42–43 pounds, 43–44 inches	Generally prefers play with other children Becomes competitive Shows evidence of responsibility and guilt

BIBLIOGRAPHY

ABDEL-GHANY, MOHAMED, "Evaluation of Household Diets by the Index of Nutritional Quality," *J. Nutr. Educ.*, vol. 10, April–June 1978.

ABRAHAM, S., G. COLLING, and M. NORSDIECK, "Relationship of Childhood Weight State to Morbidity in Adults," *HSMHA Health Repo.*, 86 (1971), 273.

ABRAMS, C.A.L., et al., "Hazards of Over-concentrated Milk Formula," *J. Amer. Med. Assoc.*, 232 (1975), 1126.

AITKEN, F.C., and F.E. HYTTEN, "Infant Feeding: Comparison of Breast and Artificial Feeding," *Nutr. Abstr. Rev.*, 30 (1960), 341.

ALLEN, K. EILEEN, *Mainstreaming in Early Childhood Education*. Albany, N.Y.: Delmar Publishers, Inc., 1980.

American Academy of Pediatrics, *Pediatric Nutrition Handbook*, Evanston, Ill.: American Academy of Pediatrics, 1979.

_____, *Recommendations for Day Care Centers for Infants and Children*. Evanston: Ill.: American Academy of Pediatrics, 1980.

ANDERSON, T.A., and S.J. FOMAN, "Commercially Prepared Infant Cereals: Nutritional Considerations," *J. Pediat.*, 78 (1971), 788.

_____, "Commercially Prepared Strained and Junior Foods for Infants," *J. Amer. Dietet. Assoc.*, 58 (1971), 520.

ANSELMO, S., "Nutritional Partnership Between Day Care Center and Home," *J. Nutr. Educ.*, vol. 7, 1975.

BARCUS, F.E., "Weekend Commercial Children's Television—1975." Action for Children's Television. Newtonville, Mass.: 1975.

BERG, A., "Crisis in Infant Feeding Practices," *Nutr. Today*, 12, no. 1, 18.

BETTELHEIM, BRUNO, "Child Rearing." Annual Editions, Readings in Human Development. Guilford, Conn.: Dushkin Publishing Group, 1973–1974.

BEYER, N.R., and P.M. MORRIS, "Food Attitudes and Snacking Patterns of Young Children," *J. Nutr. Educ.*, 6 (1974), 131.

BIRCH, L.L., "Dimensions of Preschool Children's Food Preferences," *J. Nutr. Educ.*, 11 (1979), 77–80.

BRONFENBRENNER, URIE, "Is Early Intervention Effective?" *A Report on Longitudinal Evaluations of Preschool Programs,* vol. II, 1974. Washington, D.C.: Office of Child Development, U.S. Department of Health, Education, and Welfare.

BURT, J.V., and A.A. HERTZLER, "Parental Influences on the Child's Food Preferences," *J. Nutr. Educ.,* 10 (1978), 127-28.

CALIENDO, M., and DIVA SANJUR, "The Dietary Status of Preschool Children: An Ecological Approach." *J. Nutr. Educ.,* vol. 10, April-June 1978.

CHANG, ALBERT, and MARYANN SAFFOLD, "Nutrition in Family Day Care Homes," *J. Nutr. Ed.,* 12 (1980), 146-147.

Committee on Nutrition: American Academy of Pediatrics, "Commentary on Breast Feeding and Infant Formulas," *Pediatrics,* 57 (1976), 278-85.

———,"Iron-Fortified Formulas," *Pediatrics,* 47 (1971), 786.

———,"Iron Supplementation for Infants," *Pediatrics,* 58 (1976), 765.

———,"Salt Intake and Eating Patterns of Infants and Children in Relation to Blood Pressure," *Pediatrics,* 53 (1974), 115.

COPELAND, RICHARD, *How Young Children Learn Mathematics,* New York: Macmillan, Inc., 1979.

COTT, ALLEN, "Megavitamins: The Orthomolecular Approach to Behavioral Disorders and Learning Disabilities," *Acad. Therapy,* vol. 7, no. 3, Spring 1972.

CRAVIOTO, J., and B. ROBLES, "Evolution of Adaptive Abilities and Motor Behavior During Rehabilitation from Kwashiorkor," *Amer. J. Orthopsychiatry,* 35 (1965), 448-49.

DAVIS, C.M., "Self-selection of Diets by Newly Weaned Infants," *Amer. J. Dis. Child.,* 46 (1964), 743.

DELICARDIE, M.S., and H.G. BIRCH, "Nutrition, Growth, and Neurointegrative Development: An Experimental and Ecologic Study," *Pediatrics,* vol. 38, 1966.

DWYER, J.T., et al., "The New Vegetarians," *J. Amer. Dietet. Assoc.,* 62 (1973), 503-509.

———,"The New Vegetarians: The Natural High?" *J. Amer. Dietet. Assoc.,* 65 (1974), 529-36.

DYKES, M.H.M., and P. MEIER, "Ascorbic Acid and the Common Cold: Evaluation of Its Efficacy and Toxicity," *J. Amer. Med. Assoc.,* 231 (1975), 1073-1079.

ENDRES, J.B., and R.E. ROCKWELL, *Food, Nutrition, and the Young Child,* St. Louis: The C.V. Mosby Company, 1980.

EPPRIGHT, E.S., et al., "Eating Behavior of Preschool Children," *J. Nutr. Educ.,* Summer 1969.

"Fast-Food Chains; Ratings of Meals, *Consumer Reports,* September 1979, pp. 508-13.

FDA Consumer, Department of Health and Human Services, U.S. Government Printing Office, 79-2118, 1976, 1980.

FOMAN, S.J., *Infant Nutrition* (2nd ed.). Philadelphia: W.B. Saunders Company, 1974.

FOMAN, S.J., and T.A. ANDERSON, *Practices of Low-Income Families in Feeding Infants and Small Children with Particular Attention to Cultural Subgroups.* Rockville, Md.: U.S. Department of Health, Education and Welfare, Health Services and Medical Health Administration, Maternal and Child Health Service, 1972.

FOMAN, S.J., et al., "Acceptance of Unsalted Strained Foods by Normal Infants," *J. Pediat.,* 76 (1970), 242.

————,*Prevention of Iron Deficiency Anemia in Nutritional Disorders of Children, Prevention, Screening, and Follow-Up,* U.S. Department of Health, Education and Welfare, PHS Publication No. (HSA) 77-5104. Washington, D.C.: U.S. Government Printing Office, 1977.

————,*Recommendations for Feeding Normal Infants,* DHEW Publication No. (HSA) 79-5108. Washington, D.C.: U.S. Government Printing Office, 1979.

FONOSCH, G., and E.F. KVITKA, *Meal Management.* New York: Canfield Press, 1978.

Food and Nutrition Board, National Research Council, *Recommended Dietary Allowance* (9th ed.). Washington, D.C.: National Academy of Science, 1979.

Food and Nutrition Service, *Child Care Food Program,* FNS-154m. Washington, D.C.: U.S. Department of Agriculture, 1976.

GALLENDER, DEMOR, *Teaching Eating and Toileting Skills to the MultiHandicapped in the School Setting.* Springfield, Ill.: Charles C Thomas, Publisher, 1980.

GARDNER, J.B., "A Burger Battle with Everything," *U.S. News and World Report,* November 8, 1982.

GILLIAM, THOMAS B., "Children's Sedentary Habits," *U.S.A. Today,* October 1981.

GREENWALDT, E., et al., "The Onset of Sleeping Through the Night in Infancy: Relation to Introduction of Solid Food in the Diet, Birth Weight, and Position in the Family," *Pediat.,* 26 (1960), 667.

GUSSOW, J., "Counternutritional Messages of TV Ads Aimed at Children," *J. Nutr. Educ.,* 4 (1972), 48.

GYORGY, P., "Protective Effects of Human Milk in Experimental Staphylococcal Infections," *Science,* 137 (1962), 48.

HIRSCH, J., "Studies of Adipose Tissue in Man," *Amer. J. Clin. Nutr.,* vol. 8, 1960.

HERBERT-JACKSON, E., M. W. CROSS, and T. RISLEY, "Evaluating the Folklore about Young Children's Eating." Abstract of paper presented to the Society for Nutrition Education, July 12, 1976.

HYMES, J.L., JR., *Effective Home School Relations.* Southern California Association for the Education of Young Children, 1974.

_____, *Involving Parents in Children's Learning, A Handbook for Teachers.* Whittier, Calif.: Pacific Oaks College, n.d.

_____, Project Head Start. Parents Are Needed. Suggestions on Parent Participation in Child Development Centers, No. 6, Washington, D.C.: U.S. Department of Health, Education, and Welfare.

KAMII, C., *Number in Preschool and Kindergarten: Educational Implications of Piaget's Theory.* Washington, D.C.: National Association for the Education of Young Children, 1982.

KEOUGH, C., "Rating Those Food Additives," *Organic Gardening,* February 1980.

KNITTLE, J.L., "Obesity in Childhood: A Problem in Adipose Tissue Cellular Development," *J. Pediatr.,* 6 (1972), 1048-1059.

LAPPE, F.M., *Diet for a Small Planet.* New York: Ballentine Books, Inc., 1973.

LECOS, C., "For Food Labels, Better Read; Better Fed," *FDA Consumer,* October, 1982, pp. 8-11.

LEHMANN, P., "Food Additives: A Double-Edged Sword," *Science Quest,* April 1980.

LODA, FRANK, "The Health of Children in Day Care," in *Perspectives on Infant Day Care,* eds. Richard Elardo and Betty Dagan. Little Rock, Ark.: Southern Association on Children Under Six (SACUS), 1976.

LOWENBERG, M.E., "Food Preferences of Young Children," *J. Amer. Dietet. Assoc.,* 24 (1948), 430.

MAIRS, P.; *Making Baby Food.* Ames, Iowa: Cooperative Extension Service, Iowa State University, 1978.

MAIRS, P. and C. CARLSON, *Feeding Your Baby.* Ames, Iowa: Cooperative Extension Service, Iowa State University, 1978.

Maternal and Child Health Service, *Nutrition and Feeding of Infants and Children under Three in Group Day Care.* Washington, D.C.: U.S. Government Printing Office, 1971.

McWILLIAMS, MARGARET, *Nutrition for the Growing Years,* New York: John Wiley & Sons, Inc. 1980.

LANDAW, S.A., and F.A. OSKI, "Iron Sufficiency in Breastfed Infants and the Availability of Iron from Human Milk," *Pediatrics,* 58 (1976), 686.

MENDELOFF, A.I., "Dietary Fiber and Human Health," *N. Engl. J. Med.,* 297 (1977), 811.

MEYER, H., "Breast Feeding in the United States," *Clin. Pediat.,* 7 (1968), 708.

MEYER, H.F., *Infant Foods and Feeding Practice.* Springfield, Ill.: Charles C Thomas, Publisher, 1960.

MOOSBERG, H.O.; "Obesity in Children: A Clinical Prognostical Investigation," *Acta Pediatr. Acan.* 35, suppl. no. 2, 1948.

Nutrition Foundation, "Overfeeding in First Year of Life," *Nutr. Review,* 31 (1973), 116.

OWENS, G.M., et al., "A Study of Nutritional Status in Preschool Children in the United States, 1968-1970," *Pediatrics,* 53 (1974), 597.

PAGE, L., and E. PHIPARD, *Essential of a Adequate Diet: Facts for Nutritional Programs,* USDA, Home Econ. Res. Rep. No. 3, Washington, D.C.: U.S. Government Printing Office, 1957.

PHILLIPS, BEVERLY K. and KATHRYN K. KOLASA, "Vegetable Preferences of Preschoolers in Day Care," *J. Nutr. Educ.,* vol. 12, October-December 1980.

PHILLIPS, DORIS E., and MARY BASS, "Use of Food and Nutrition Knowledge by Mothers of Preschool Children," *Journal of Nutrition Education,* vol. 10, April-June 1978.

PIAGET, J., *Judgement and Reasoning in the Child.* New York: Humanities Press, Inc., 1964.

PUYAU, F.A., and L.P. HAMPTON, "Infant Feeding Practices, 1966. Salt Content of Modern Diets." *Amer. J. Dis. Child.,* 111 (1966), 370.

Select Committees on Nutrition and Human Needs, *Dietary Goals for the United States,* Washington, D.C.: U.S. Government Printing Office, December 1977.

SMICIKLAS-WRIGHT, HELEN, FLORENCE PETERSEN, and DONALD PETERS, "Day Care Nutrition Programs and Children's Home Diets." *Child Care Quarterly,* Spring 1979, pp. 47-58.

SPEER, F., "Management of Food Allergy," *Allergy and Immunology in Children,* eds. F. Speer and R.J. Dockhor. Springfield, Ill.: Charles C Thomas, Publisher, 1973.

STEPHENSON, M.G., "Making Food Labels More Useful and Informative," *Aging,* September-October 1980, pp. 29-32.

STOKES, S.J., "Decoding Food Labels," *Essence,* May 1981, pp. 138-41.

SWEENY, M.E., and M.F. BRECKENRIDGE, *How to Feed Children in Nursery Schools.* Detroit, Mich.: Merrill-Palmer School, 1951.

TIATZ, L.S., "Obesity in Practice: Infantile Obesity," *Pediatr. Clin. North Am.,* 24 (1977), 107.

TURNER, M.D., and J.S. TURNER, *Making Your Own Baby Food,* New York: Workman Publishing Co., 1976.

WANAMAKER, N., K. HEARN, and S. RICHARZ, *More Than Graham Crackers: Nutrition Education and Food Preparation with Young Children.* Washington, D.C.: National Association for the Education of Young Children (NAEYC), 1979.

WILLIAMS, S., A. HENNEMAN, and H. FOX, "Contributions of Food Service Programs in Preschool Centers to Children's Nutritional Needs," *J. Amer. Dietet. Assoc.,* 71 (1977), 612.

WINICK, MYRON, and P. RUSSO, "The Effects of Severe Early Malnutrition of Cellular Growth of the Human Brain," *Pediatric Research,* 3 (1969), 181-84.

WYDEN, BARBARA, "Growth: 45 Crucial Months," *Life,* December 1971.

INDEX